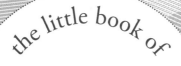

the little book of

REST

100+ Ways to
Relax and Restore Your
Mind, Body, and Soul

Stephanie Thomas

Adams Media
New York London Toronto Sydney New Delhi

To Lady and Bo, the best dogs in the world—and the perfect examples of how to relax and enjoy every day.

Adams media

Adams Media
An Imprint of Simon & Schuster, Inc.
100 Technology Center Drive
Stoughton, Massachusetts 02072

First Adams Media hardcover edition November 2022

ADAMS MEDIA and colophon are trademarks of Simon & Schuster.

For information about special discounts for bulk purchases, please contact Simon & Schuster Special Sales at 1-866-506-1949 or business@simonandschuster.com.

The Simon & Schuster Speakers Bureau can bring authors to your live event. For more information or to book an event contact the Simon & Schuster Speakers Bureau at 1-866-248-3049 or visit our website at www.simonspeakers.com.

Interior design by Michelle Kelly
Images © 123RF/bwise

Manufactured in China

10 9 8 7 6 5 4 3 2 1

Library of Congress Control Number: 2022935527

ISBN 978-1-5072-1939-3
ISBN 978-1-5072-1940-9 (ebook)

contents

chapter 1: physical 13

chapter 2: mental

chapter 3: emotional 107

chapter 4: spiritual 151

*introduction

When most people hear the word "rest," they immediately think of taking naps or sleeping. Although these are effective ways to unwind, this book will show you there are many more ways to incorporate relaxation into your day that don't involve sleep.

The Little Book of Rest is intended to shift your mindset from viewing rest and relaxation as privileges you can take part in only after you have completed *everything else* on your never-ending to-do list, to realizing that rest and relaxation need to be a priority because they're essential for your overall health and well-being. Healthy living requires taking care of yourself as a whole—mind, body, and spirit. Throughout this book, you'll learn the importance of taking time to rest and relax and how beneficial and necessary rest and relaxation are for healthy living. You'll also discover more than one hundred simple activities you can do all day long to experience more peace and tranquility in your life.

Adding restful and relaxing activities into your day doesn't have to be just another tedious task on your to-do list. Unlike other self-care activities that require large amounts of time or energy, the activities in this book are simple, are enjoyable, and require minimal effort—they're things you'll genuinely look forward to!

The Little Book of Rest has four chapters: physical, mental, emotional, and spiritual. The activities range from different forms of light physical activity such as foam rolling and restorative yoga, to meditative and mindfulness practices such as deep breathing and coloring. You'll also find healing emotional release practices such as allowing yourself to cry, screaming with a friend, and releasing judgment, as well as enlightening spiritual practices such as spending time alone, spending time in silence, and spending time in prayer.

As you flip through the following pages, choose your favorite activities from each chapter, and start taking some much-needed time to rest and relax!

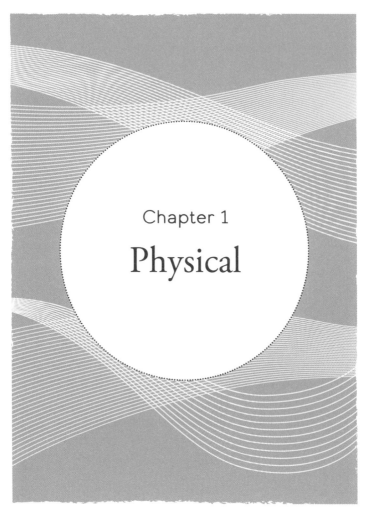

Chapter 1
Physical

Learning to properly rest your physical body is crucial to your well-being. Rest does not necessarily mean doing nothing. The activities in this chapter will give you the opportunity to explore various forms of nonstrenuous physical activities such as walking and stretching, helpful practices for being more in tune with your body such as tai chi and slow flow yoga, and simple tools for relaxing and healing your body such as acupressure and restorative yoga.

Choose the activities that you believe will be the most enjoyable and beneficial for you and give them a try. You'll quickly realize that not all physical activities deplete your energy; some physical activities such as walking in nature and starting a new workout routine may actually boost your energy and make you feel even better than taking a nap would.

A sense of ease should guide your approach to physical activity. By engaging in restorative and replenishing types of movement, you facilitate healing and recovery in your body. When you move through life with ease and prioritize rest and relaxation, positive energy will fill every aspect of your life.

Try Foam Rolling

Would you like a do-it-yourself massage? Foam rolling, known as self-myofascial release, helps release tension in your muscles, reduces inflammation and soreness, and increases joint flexibility. In fact, this activity can relax your muscles so much that you'll feel as if you've just had a full body massage, leaving you better able to rest.

This muscle relaxation tool is typically cylindrical and made with dense foam. Foam rollers are available in various shapes and sizes, as well as different degrees of firmness so you can decide how intense you want the rollers to feel. You can find them in the fitness or sporting goods section at your local store or online.

A few tips:

* Be gentle at first. Start with light pressure by using your hands to lift your body weight over the roller, instead of fully sinking into it.
* Roll on a muscle for at least thirty seconds. When you reach a painful or sore area, hold it there for a few seconds and slowly increase the pressure for ten seconds.
* Some important places to target are your legs, glutes, and upper back.

* After you've completed your rolling session, drink plenty of water, and stay hydrated throughout the day.

Start your foam rolling practice by foam rolling for ten minutes once per week. If you enjoy it, do it as frequently as you like.

Practice the Legs-Up-the-Wall Pose

Legs-Up-the-Wall is a restorative yoga pose that focuses on relaxing and releasing tension. The soothing nature of this pose elicits the relaxation response, a neurological response that pulls you out of "fight-or-flight" mode and brings you into a state of "rest and digest." In this state, anxiety and stress are reduced, immunity is strengthened, muscle tension is released, and a feeling of general well-being envelops you.

To practice the Legs-Up-the-Wall Pose:

1. Find a bare wall and sit with your right side against the wall. Then, slowly lie back and rotate your body as you swing your legs up against the wall so that the bottoms of your feet are facing the ceiling.
2. Scoot in toward the wall so that your tailbone is as close to the wall as possible. Let your legs relax into the wall, keeping a slight bend in your knees if your hamstrings are tight.
3. If you prefer a little more cushioning, place a folded blanket under your head.
4. Rest with your arms by your sides, palms up.
5. Completely relax your legs and the rest of your body, and just breathe slowly for five to ten minutes.

Take a Relaxing Bubble Bath

A bubble bath might sound like a luxury, but it is a simple way to relax your body and mind. The warmth and weight of the water will make you feel like you're in a safe cocoon. Adding bubbles to your bath will bring out your inner child and playful spirit. Simply lying back and relaxing in a bathtub can help clear your mind of worries and stressors from the day.

Not only do baths help you relax mentally, but they also are beneficial to your physical body. Soaking in warm water can reduce inflammation, relieve muscle pain, and alleviate tension in your body. Adding Epsom salts or essential oils can also help with this!

You don't need anything fancy to make a bubble bath feel like a special treat, and why not treat yourself regularly? Just use your favorite bubble bath mix, bath bomb, or bath salts and enjoy the soothing benefits. While relaxing in the tub, you can listen to calming music or read a couple of chapters in a good book.

Bubble baths can quickly become part of your evening routine and will give you something to look forward to throughout a stressful day.

Take a Silent Walk in Nature

Have you ever taken a walk and just focused on the multiple sounds around you? Taking a walk outside can feel even more relaxing than a nap! It can be remarkably soothing to your mind to simply listen to the sounds of nature. Do your best to be present and mindful during your walk. When you catch your mind wandering or notice that you are thinking about what's next on your to-do list, don't judge yourself, but just gently guide your mind back to the sounds. Name all the sounds you can hear right now in this present moment: leaves rustling in the trees, birds singing, bees buzzing around, waves crashing, the soothing sound of water flowing down a stream, and so on. Focusing on the various sounds you encounter on your walk will allow your mind and body to relax and decompress from the day.

You don't have to go to a park, a beach, or a wooded trail to enjoy a walk in nature. Just find a safe place to go for a walk, make sure your phone is on silent, and spend at least ten minutes walking and enjoying the present moment and all the beauty nature has to offer.

Start an Herb Garden

Gardening is not only a great activity for boosting your mood, but also an amazing skill to learn. Planting seeds is a relaxing activity on its own—studies have shown that having your hands in the soil increases serotonin levels. If you complete this activity outdoors, you will further increase your serotonin levels from receiving the benefits of the sunshine and fresh air. Serotonin is a hormone released by the brain that promotes a sense of calm, well-being, and happiness.

An herb garden is a great way to get into gardening because it doesn't take much effort and you don't need a large amount of space. An herb garden can also be planted inside or outside so you can start in any season.

You can start growing herbs from seeds or use transplants. Herbs can be planted in separate small pots, or you can combine a few herbs in one large pot. To begin, you just need a few seeds or transplants, some potting soil, and a pot or two. Some versatile herbs you can start with are peppermint, basil, thyme, sage, oregano, rosemary, and lavender.

Watching the herbs sprout and grow feels so rewarding, and eventually you'll have your own homegrown herbs to add to your healthy meals!

Drink Chamomile Tea

Consider adding chamomile tea to your nightly routine. This ancient herbal tea is known for its calming effects. Sipping on chamomile tea about an hour before you are ready to go to sleep is a very relaxing way to wind down and prepare for sleep. Drinking chamomile tea also enhances the quality of sleep because it contains antioxidants that promote drowsiness. In addition, this tea is rich in antioxidants that are known to decrease inflammation and reduce the risk of chronic disease.

To enjoy the many benefits of chamomile tea, start by bringing 8 ounces of water to a boil. Then place the chamomile tea bag in the water (or add the chamomile leaves to a tea ball), letting it steep for about five minutes. Once the tea is ready, add a little lemon juice or honey and stir.

Sit down, relax, and slowly sip the tea. In between sips, take long, deep breaths to assist with relaxation. Inhaling the aroma of the tea can also help you feel calmer. Be sure to make your cup of tea about an hour before bed so you can truly experience a more relaxed state and more restful sleep.

Practice Restorative Yoga
with a Bolster

Practicing restorative yoga weekly can help boost your mental and physical well-being. It provides a soothing effect on the nervous system and can help your sleep feel more restful.

Restorative yoga is quite different from other yoga forms because of its slow style, its emphasis on recovery, and the way in which you support your body in a pose, relax into it, and stay in the same pose for several minutes (up to ten minutes).

Often, yoga bolsters are used for support. They are large, firm pillows that come in different shapes and sizes. When you use a bolster in restorative yoga, you're able to perform certain poses more safely and comfortably. Using a bolster allows you to feel stretched, released, and relaxed. You can find these pillows in the fitness section at your local store or online.

Following the guidance of a yoga teacher when you first begin restorative yoga is an excellent practice. You can search for restorative yoga on *YouTube* and follow the teacher's step-by-step instructions.

Yoga practice is a sacred time to just be with yourself and listen to what your body tells you. When you hold a pose for a long time, you will be able to connect with yourself on a deeper level.

Relax in a Hammock

Just the thought of lying in a hammock can be peaceful. You don't need to go to a tropical location to enjoy relaxing in a hammock! All you need are two large trees close to each other in your yard, or if you only have open space without trees, you can buy a hammock stand that will allow you to place your hammock anywhere you want! Hammocks come in many different styles and materials, so be sure to pick the one that is most comfortable for you. You can find thousands to explore online.

While you're lying in a hammock is a great time to practice meditation, listen to music, or read a book. You can even cuddle up with a loved one and enjoy the peacefulness together. Be present by feeling the gentle rocking of the hammock, smelling the fresh air around you, and listening to the sounds of nature. Lying in a hammock is also a wonderful time to take a nap! Did you know that sleeping in a hammock is good for you? It doesn't put pressure on your spine and helps your body fully relax. So, the next time you lie in a hammock, don't be afraid to allow yourself to fall asleep.

Try a Hot Stone Massage

Getting a hot stone massage not only feels like a relaxing treat, but also provides numerous health benefits such as releasing tension in tight muscles and soft tissues, reducing anxiety and stress, and deepening sleep.

Although using rocks during massage may not sound calming at first, this healing treatment will leave you feeling relaxed and rejuvenated. It should be easy to find a local hot stone massage service as they are available at most wellness spas.

During a hot stone massage, the massage therapist will place flat, hot stones on various parts of your body. The stones typically used are made from a volcanic rock called basalt. This rock, normally heated to around 140°F, is great at retaining heat, making it useful for hot stone massages.

The hot stones can be placed on your stomach, hands, back, chest, and even feet and face. The massage therapist may simply hold the hot stones while kneading in a Swedish massage style.

This unique massage style will benefit you if you are experiencing any muscle aches, anxiety, or trouble sleeping. If you have chronic conditions, be sure to seek approval from your doctor before trying a hot stone massage.

Book a Custom Facial at a Local Spa

What feels more relaxing than getting a facial? Not only are you doing something amazing to take care of your skin, but you also are dedicating time to pure mental bliss. When you get a facial, it feels so soothing that it can bring you into a meditative state. During a facial, you can expect your skin to be cleansed, exfoliated, and massaged. Because everyone's skin is so different, it's best to get a "custom" facial at a local spa so that the esthetician can focus on your skin's specific needs.

Getting a facial provides you with a state of relaxation, renews your skin, boosts your mood, and gives you a beautiful glow, while continuing to offer benefits long after the "feel good" factor has worn off. A facial is well known for relieving stress and soothing the mind. In addition, facials assist in detoxification, as well as removing excess fluid from your body, allowing your skin to achieve optimal health, and encouraging the regeneration of cells in your skin. Taking good care of your skin is about more than just improving your appearance; it is all about keeping the largest organ in your body healthy. Why not enjoy the experience?

Use a Lavender Pillow Spray

Lavender is one of the most relaxing scents you can find. This fragrant herb has been used as a soothing aromatic for a long time! Lavender has many calming capabilities, and studies have shown that lavender not only helps you fall asleep faster and remain asleep longer but also improves the overall quality of sleep. Upon waking up, you feel well rested and refreshed when utilizing lavender.

Therefore, a lavender pillow spray could be a great addition to your nightly bedtime routine. Before getting into bed, lightly mist your pillow, sheets, and/or pajamas with the lavender spray, and then climb into bed and peacefully drift off to sleep.

Lavender pillow sprays are easy to find in stores; just look for one that is all-natural and made with 100 percent pure essential oils.

If you would rather make your own spray, you'll need:

* Eight ounces distilled water
* Five drops pure lavender oil
* Small spray bottle

Simply combine the water and drops of oil in the bottle and shake well. Shake the bottle before every use.

If you don't like the idea of spraying your pillow and then laying your face on it, you can achieve the same results using an essential oil diffuser.

Take Five Minutes to Stretch Every Day

We often don't take time to stretch. This is the ultimate form of self-care and rest you can give your muscles. Your muscles are constantly working for you, and if you don't take the time to stretch them, they will get extremely tight. Tight muscles can lead to potential injury and reduced range of movement. You may even experience constant discomfort or chronic pain in your body from a lack of mobility and flexibility.

Try a daily five-minute stretch when you first wake up, before bed, or anytime you choose! Search for "simple stretches" online and try a variety of them to implement a daily practice.

Some examples of simple stretches:

* Sit on the floor with your legs out in front of you and lean forward, reaching toward your toes, feeling the stretch in your legs.
* Stand up straight and lean slightly to one side with your arms stretched out, pointed in the direction you are leaning, and then switch sides, feeling the stretch in your sides.

✱ Sit in a chair facing forward; then twist your body to the right, grabbing the back of the chair as you twist, and then switch sides, feeling the stretch in your back.

Eat Dark Chocolate

Not only is eating dark chocolate relaxing, but it also is surprisingly good for you. It's true! You can now enjoy dark chocolate in moderation without feeling guilty because it has many health benefits.

Dark chocolate is loaded with nutrients like fiber, copper, iron, manganese, and magnesium. Chocolate in its purest form contains powerful antioxidants and several compounds that work with the chemistry of your brain to promote feeling good. Chocolate also contains tryptophan, an amino acid that is the precursor for serotonin. Therefore, when you consume chocolate, you experience an increase in serotonin, which produces feelings of calm, well-being, and happiness.

For you to fully experience the benefits of dark chocolate, it's essential to consider the type of dark chocolate you're buying and what is included in the ingredient list. Look for dark chocolate that contains at least 70 percent cocoa. The ingredient label must have cacao butter, the natural, healthy fat that comes from cacao beans. Look for chocolate bars with five ingredients or fewer, and stay away from bars that include ingredients you cannot pronounce.

Be mindful of how much chocolate you consume. Remember, it is good for you *in moderation*. Most importantly, enjoy!

Use an Acupressure Mat

Acupressure, a form of Traditional Chinese Medicine, is a healing technique that uses different pressure points on the body to promote relaxation and wellness and treat diseases. This practice applies the same principles as acupuncture, just without the needles!

To reap the benefits of acupressure without going to an acupressure practitioner, you can purchase an acupressure mat and practice this healing technique on your own. Acupressure mats help you experience similar benefits to the ones achieved from acupressure or acupuncture sessions with a professional.

Acupressure mats are also known as "beds of needles," as the spikes on the mats are sharp and may cause discomfort at first, but don't let that keep you from trying! The benefits are worth the initial pain. Since there are multiple spikes on the mat, it stimulates many acupressure points at once. Using an acupressure mat can help alleviate headaches, neck pain, back pain, tight or sore muscles, and stress. The mat has a calming effect, signaling to your nervous system that you are safe and secure.

The first time you use an acupressure mat, you may need a bit of time to adjust, but most people end up really enjoying it with regular use!

Practice Tai Chi

Originally a Chinese tradition, tai chi is a form of relaxing, meditative exercise for people of all fitness levels and is also known as a movement meditation. Tai chi is a martial arts–style practice with slow movements and deep breathing. Tai chi is a gentle physical practice, but it can also benefit your mind. Compared to other forms of exercise, it is quite relaxing.

Tai chi has many benefits, including:

* Improving cognition
* Lessening anxiety
* Decreasing depression
* Improving quality of sleep
* Improving posture and body alignment
* Increasing flexibility and mobility in muscles
* Increasing body awareness and reducing the risk of falling due to imbalance

What should you do once you decide to give tai chi a try? Here are some tips:

* Look for a local gym or studio that offers beginner tai chi classes.

* If you would prefer to be guided one-on-one, ask the teacher if personal sessions are available.
* Watch tai chi classes or single movements on *YouTube*.
* With an instructor's permission, consider observing an in-person session.
* If you are not Chinese, don't be intimidated by the unfamiliar directions and language. It's all about relaxing and enjoying the present moment. Learning more about another culture is a plus!

Take Your Dog for a Walk

What's better than a relaxing walk in nature? Bringing your dog along! Just having your dog around lowers your stress and makes you feel more relaxed by reducing the levels of cortisol in your body. You can relieve feelings of loneliness, stress, anxiety, and depression by taking your dog for regular walks.

Going for a walk sparks joy and curiosity in dogs, and they eagerly explore everything they can, thoroughly enjoying the adventure. Simply witnessing their joy and enthusiasm for life can be joyful for you as well. Make sure that when your dog stops to smell the roses, you do too!

On the other hand, the slower pace of a nature trail is incredibly calming, and you can free your mind when there is less hustle and bustle around. If you stop to take a small break during your walk, notice how your dog carelessly sprawls out on the ground beneath you and basks happily in the warm sun pouring down. Allow yourself to do the same for a few minutes and really soak in the tranquility of the moment. It is so peaceful and relaxing to feel the warmth of the sun on your face while mindfully sitting in stillness.

Take a Yoga Class at a Local Studio

One of the most beneficial reasons to practice yoga at a local studio is for the relaxing environment. Many yoga studios include dim lighting, gentle music, and calming scents from incense or essential oils—all of which encourage students to maintain their mindfulness. With electronic devices prohibited, there should be little opportunity for distractions when you are practicing at the studio. It is your time to focus on yourself and relax.

Going to a local yoga class allows you to ask questions or get one-on-one guidance from the teacher. The great thing about being in a class setting is that your instructor will help you achieve the proper form and reduce your likelihood of injury. You'll also be able to learn different types of yoga practices that you might not be exposed to at home or online.

Attending a class will give you a sense of community and belonging and give you the opportunity to meet like-minded people with similar interests. Not only will you be doing good things for your body, but you'll also be making friends who also enjoy the wonderful benefits of relaxation, mindfulness, and health and wellness.

Eat Well-Balanced Meals

Eating a healthy, well-balanced diet can improve concentration and focus, helping you feel well rested and ready to tackle anything on your to-do list. Food is energy, and it directly affects your energy levels. A well-balanced diet that provides vitamins, minerals, and nutrients is essential to keep your body and mind strong and healthy.

Eating healthy provides benefits such as disease prevention, positive energy, restful sleep, maintenance of a healthy weight, and improved brain function. Having a balanced diet will ensure the body gets the proper quantities of carbohydrates, fats, proteins, vitamins, and minerals.

You might wonder, what exactly makes up a well-balanced meal? If you eat three meals a day, aim for each meal to include balanced portions of all macronutrients: proteins (for example, chicken, eggs), carbohydrates (such as brown rice, sweet potato), and fats (for example, avocado, olive oil, and so on).

One of the first steps toward eating a healthy, well-balanced diet is to become aware of your thoughts and feelings around food, eating, and weight. Start a food journal and write down what you eat every day and how you feel before, during, and afterward. You will notice eating patterns and how they affect your energy, sleep, and mood.

Try a Hot-Shower Meditation

One of the most relaxing things you can do after a stressful day is taking a long, hot shower. The hot water increases your body temperature and relieves the tension in your muscles, especially in your shoulders, neck, and back. When you soothe and loosen tight muscles, it relaxes you not only physically, but also mentally. This can prepare your body for a peaceful sleep.

Taking a hot shower first thing in the morning can also be very soothing and help you begin your day feeling calmer and more relaxed.

Here's a quick and easy shower meditation you can practice as you wash:

To begin, stand under the running water and for about a minute just focus on the feeling of the hot water running down your body. Taking slow, deep breaths in and out, mindfully focus on the soothing feeling of the water. Then proceed to wash your hair, face, and body as you always do, only this time you are consciously imagining that as you wash yourself, any stress and tension you feel and any negative energy you've been carrying around are also being washed away and are disappearing down the drain with the water and soap.

Take a Slow Flow Yoga Class

As the name suggests, slow flow yoga is simply a slower version of regular-paced Vinyasa (or flow) yoga classes. In this type of class, you will spend more time focusing on your breathing and holding each posture. During slow flow, yogis use more mindfulness and attention when coming in and out of poses, which is a great time for beginners to explore each pose. All levels of yogis experience greater calm and less feeling of being overwhelmed when attending a slow flow class.

Slow flow yoga is an excellent style of yoga to perform close to bedtime because it soothes your body from the stressors of the day and helps your mind unwind. It's so relaxing that you may want to add it to your nightly routine a few times a week! Many yoga studios offer slow flow classes in the evening since it is such a great way to unwind and relax after a long day. If you don't wish to attend a local yoga studio, search for slow flow yoga on *YouTube* and enjoy a few classes from the comfort of home.

Give Yourself a Foot Massage

A foot massage isn't just super-relaxing, but it also provides many health benefits such as improving circulation, reducing tension and stress, easing pain, and stimulating muscles. How can rubbing your feet do all that? There are thousands of nerve endings in each of your feet, and when these are stimulated during a foot massage, it activates your nervous system, increasing the number of feel-good brain chemicals (endorphins) being released.

Massaging your own feet is easy to do! Here's a simple technique you can follow:

1. Sit in a chair or on your bed with your feet on the floor. Lift one of your feet up and rest it on the opposite thigh.
2. Put some lotion or massage oil in your hands and start massaging your heel, arch, and toes, rubbing the lotion or oil into the skin as you massage your entire foot.
3. Use simple massage techniques, like kneading your foot with your knuckles and pressing your thumb to make small circles. To stretch the muscles of your toes, slowly push each toe forward and back and massage each toe in a circular motion.
4. Repeat the process on the other foot.

Try a Do-It-Yourself Home Facial

Giving yourself a facial at home is an easy and decadent way to relax and unwind after a long day. Here is a quick and easy method that will get you feeling relaxed and pampered in no time.

To fully embrace the spa experience, start by making cucumber water the night before. Cut up a cucumber and infuse it in a large pitcher of water. Refrigerate the cucumber water overnight. On the day of your home facial, drink at least one cup of the cucumber water before you begin your facial. This will hydrate your skin from the inside out and enhance your natural healthy glow.

1. Gently massage some cleanser into your skin in small circular motions. Rinse with warm water.
2. Rub an exfoliator or a face scrub gently across your skin to remove dead skin cells and uncover your natural radiance. Rinse with warm water.
3. Use your preferred face mask (based on your skin's unique needs) as directed on the package. For the final time, rinse your face with warm water, and then pat gently with a soft towel to dry.
4. Gently massage a nighttime moisturizer into your skin to provide extra hydration throughout the night.

Prioritize Going to Bed Early

Of course sleep will help you feel relaxed, but going to bed early and waking up early are daily practices that provide countless benefits to your overall health and well-being. Keeping a consistent sleep schedule also regulates your circadian rhythm, and this leads to deeper, better-quality sleep.

Some of the benefits of implementing this daily practice are a stronger immune system, a lower risk of disease, more energy, a decrease in anxiety and depression, sharper thinking skills, increased productivity, and feeling happier in general.

To begin going to bed earlier, you will want to commit to turning off all devices at a reasonable hour, preferably an hour or so before you plan to lie down to sleep. Watching TV, scrolling on your phone, playing video games, and so on are all very stimulating activities that will make it difficult to go to sleep right after.

You will want to choose a calming activity to do before bed, such as reading (not on a device because the blue light from phones and e-readers affects your circadian rhythms), journaling, taking a hot shower, or meditating. Make your bedroom as peaceful as possible by dimming the lights and focusing on a calming activity that will allow your mind to unwind and prepare for restful sleep.

Start Your Day with a Morning Meditation

Meditation in the morning helps you feel more relaxed and better prepared to manage stressful situations as they occur throughout the day because meditation affects reactivity in the amygdala, the part of the brain that controls your stress response. A five- or ten-minute meditation in the morning will set the tone for the entire day and propel you into the day feeling grounded, supported, confident, and positive.

If you are new to meditation, you can simply sit up in your bed and, with your eyes closed, take deep, slow breaths, and focus all your attention on your breathing. Notice how the air feels as you inhale, feeling your chest expand as it fills with clean air, and then feel your chest relax as you exhale. If you notice your mind wandering to your to-do list or anything other than your breath, just gently guide it back to the feeling of the air. You can also count the inhales and exhales if this is easier. You just want to focus on something so your mind isn't doing its normal racing from one concern to another obligation, and so on.

Morning meditation with consistent practice can lead you to feel more relaxed and calm, and can benefit your mental health long-term.

Book a Blowout at a Local Salon

Remember how soothing it felt the last time someone played with your hair? Booking a blowout at a salon is a wonderful expression of self-care and oh, so relaxing! It feels amazing when someone is taking care of you and pampering you, even if you could do it yourself. Treating yourself to this "luxury" provides many benefits to your overall health and well-being. For example, human touch in this manner elicits feelings of safety and trust. More importantly, human touch releases a hormone called oxytocin, aka "the love hormone," which just makes you feel good.

Hair-blowout services tend to feel like a head massage and cause your otherwise tense facial muscles to relax. Getting your hair shampooed and blow-dried professionally is a perfect way to relax, unwind, and release any feelings of stress. The environment of a hair salon is generally welcoming, peaceful, and relaxing as well.

Having a fresh blowout also makes you feel beautiful and confident and causes your positive energy to soar. Call and book an appointment now!

Take a Yin Yoga Class

Yin yoga is a slower, more meditative style of yoga that allows you to focus inward and tune in to not only your mind but also the physical sensations of your body. Your parasympathetic nervous system is activated during this practice, which slows your heart rate and calms your body. Yin yoga encourages greater flexibility, more circulation, and better muscle recovery. This unique yoga practice targets your deep connective tissues, such as your fascia, joints, bones, and ligaments.

During yin yoga, yogis will hold yoga postures for several minutes, sometimes even up to twenty minutes in a single pose. It's imperative to focus on deep breathing in these classes, which allows you to settle even further into poses. This slow practice teaches you how to rest, be still, and be patient, even during the discomfort of staying in a posture for a prolonged period.

For yin yoga, you will need some props like blocks, blankets, and bolsters so that you can drop into postures more comfortably. Many yoga studios or fitness centers offer yin yoga, and there are many class options online as well. Try this style of yoga and it just might become your favorite way of taking some time to rest and recover.

Give Yourself a Face Massage

A face massage can be very relaxing and it's easy to give yourself one in the comfort of your own home. Not only will you feel more relaxed and rejuvenated after, but it benefits your skin by improving the appearance of your skin's texture, increasing blood flow, releasing tension in facial muscles, and relieving sinus pressure.

Take a moment to clean your face and hands before beginning. To ensure your fingers glide smoothly over your skin, apply a small amount of facial serum or moisturizer to your entire face.

When massaging your face, focus on each small area for about thirty seconds before moving on to another area. Apply firm but gentle pressure with your hands.

There are many different techniques for facial massage; try doing an online search to learn about them. Here are a few to try:

* Apply pressure to your temples by making small circles with your thumbs.
* Using a small circular motion, trace your jawline.
* Press the area under your cheekbones and slowly move your fingers outward.

* Press your fingers in the area between your eyebrows and make small circles; then slide your fingers in an upward motion on your forehead.
* Gently tap your fingertips across your face.

Use a Lavender Eye Pillow

Do you feel stressed or tired after a long day? Take a break from the world around you by leaning back and covering your eyes with a lavender-scented eye pillow. Aromatherapy eye pillows are perfect for use before bedtime or when you want to relax throughout the day. Lavender helps you relax, calms your nerves, and encourages a better night's sleep.

Eye pillows are usually weighted using rice or wheat so they can relieve tension in your forehead, jaw, cheekbones, and neck. Eye pillows aren't just for comforting fatigued eyes. When you use them, not only will your facial muscles decompress, but your mind will get a break from all the stimuli constantly around you.

If briefly chilled in the refrigerator, eye pillows can be great for relieving headaches and reducing eye puffiness and dark circles. Many eye pillows can be used hot or cold, but make sure you read the package. You can find many options to choose from online.

After you put the eye pillow on your eyes, breathe slowly and deeply as you lie back and relax into the experience. Taking at least five minutes to be still and to quiet your mind can feel challenging at first, but it gets easier with practice.

Go for a Bike Ride in Nature

Going for a bike ride on a nature trail is incredibly therapeutic for the body and mind. Biking outdoors can make you feel carefree and childlike. It allows you to let go and enjoy the present moment and all the beauty nature provides.

Aside from making sure your surroundings are clear and staying on the path, cycling does not require active thinking. It can become a form of active meditation and allow you to mentally disconnect.

Bring awareness to your legs' repetitive movements, the rate of your breath, and the air temperature around you. You will be surprised how readily your mind will clear if you focus only on these physical sensations and actions when riding.

The combination of exercise and being outdoors can be magical. Physical activity will encourage an endorphin boost, naturally making you feel good. That's why you tend to feel happier and get an energy boost after a workout. But combining a workout with being in nature is even more beneficial and is referred to as "green exercise." Green exercise increases your motivation, improves feelings of belonging and self-esteem, and reduces negative emotions. Add outdoor cycling to your workout routine to experience the rejuvenating benefits for yourself!

Use the Sauna after a Workout

Want to relax and unwind right after your workout? Try your gym's sauna! It can quickly turn your training into a spa experience. Saunas are heated rooms ranging from 150°F to 195°F (65°C to 90°C). You can stay in the sauna anywhere from five minutes up to twenty minutes, assuming you can endure the heat. Because your body will sweat significantly, you must hydrate appropriately before, during, and after using the sauna.

Through increased blood circulation and oxygen delivery to tired muscles, sauna use enhances muscle recovery. It also relieves muscle tension by allowing muscles to relax. Use this time to release anxious thoughts, reflect on your day, or practice meditation.

In addition to promoting mental and physical relaxation, a ten-minute sauna session after a workout can result in heart health benefits. High temperatures in a sauna expand blood vessels, improving circulation and lowering blood pressure.

If you are new to using a sauna, make sure to shower beforehand, wear a bathing suit or towel, and don't bring your cell phone. You can turn your sauna spa experience into a routine and enjoy it after your workouts most days of the week. You will feel refreshed and ready for whatever lies ahead!

Slow Dance with a Loved One

When is the last time you slow danced? Remember the positive feelings it evoked in you? This simple low-impact activity brings joy, love, and connection to your life. Letting your body move with the music can feel childlike, carefree, and joyous. You will also bond both emotionally and physically with your partner.

Listening to calming music while slow dancing helps you feel relaxed and tranquil. Find a playlist that brings you joy and peace. Start listening and let the music wash over you. Dancing can bring about a sense of creativity and mindfulness. Feel free to play around with some of your favorite dance moves or try some new ones!

Be in the present moment, and don't worry about what you look like. Dancing is good for your soul. If you need dance-move ideas or want to work on a particular dance, search online for step-by-step video instructions. Start by dancing with your loved one in your living room, and you might have so much fun that you will be inspired to take professional lessons or start dancing in public!

Let Your Muscles Recover

You are probably thinking, what does focusing on muscle recovery have to do with rest and relaxation?! But hear me out! I am highlighting the importance of rest from physical activity, especially if you've recently started a new workout routine!

Typically, when you begin a new workout routine, you use your muscles in new and different ways than you have in the past. This could cause slight to moderate soreness for a few days, and you may naturally feel more tired than usual. Your body is telling you that it needs to recover. Listen to your body and take time to rest. You can do this by taking extra time to stretch, practicing yoga for ten minutes, or using a foam roller.

Many people believe that you should just fight through the pain and keep working out harder and harder when working toward a fitness goal. But keep in mind the importance of listening to your body and taking time to rest or practice less strenuous activities when your body is alerting you that you are pushing it too hard.

Taking time to rest when physically active is vital to staying healthy, and a key part of this is getting enough sleep each night. Without adequate sleep, you will feel completely exhausted.

Practice Progressive Muscle Relaxation

Progressive muscle relaxation is a deep relaxation technique that teaches you how to relax your muscles by alternating between tension and relaxation in all the body's major muscle groups. By focusing on each muscle and what it feels like when tightened and relaxed, you can become more present and aware of feelings in your body.

Lie down or sit comfortably and take slow, deep breaths, allowing your body to fully relax. Begin by tightening and creating tension in your toes for about five to seven seconds. Then release the tension, causing the toes to relax. Focus on the physical sensations you are experiencing as you tighten and relax the muscles.

Work your way up your body, repeating this process for each of the major muscle groups. For example:

* On each hand and lower arm—clench your fist and tense the lower arm.
* On each lower leg and foot—point your toe and gently tense the calf muscle.
* For your abdomen—pull your abdominal muscles in tightly.

✳ For your lower forehead—frown and pull your eyebrows together.

To get the most out of this relaxation method, you will want to practice it daily. With consistent practice, you will notice yourself feeling a lot more relaxed in general.

Do a Walking Meditation

Meditation can be done anywhere, at any time, and is so relaxing. An easy way to start meditating regularly is to begin a walking meditation practice, also known as mindfulness in motion. In addition to being relaxing, this comforting practice is a great way to enhance your mood, improve digestion, and increase blood circulation.

There are a few tips to note before you begin practicing. First, choose a place to walk, either indoors or outdoors, that is free from distraction with relatively flat ground and far from traffic or crowds of people. Start each walk by taking a few deep breaths and bringing your awareness to any sensations in your body.

Feel your feet firm on the ground and acknowledge that you are always supported. As you begin to walk slowly, notice how your legs and feet move with every step. Relax your leg muscles and let your arms and hands hang freely by your sides.

Focus your attention on your breathing and any sensations you feel. As you notice thoughts coming into your awareness, let each one pass you by like a cloud in the sky. Enjoy your walking meditation for about ten to twenty minutes. If you have trouble getting in the right headspace, there are free guided walking meditations on *YouTube* and *Spotify*.

Invest In a Comfortable Pillow

Just like a quality mattress, a comfortable pillow is essential for proper rest! Your bed pillow can be the difference between a good night's sleep and waking up with a stiff neck. Sleeping with a decent pillow helps keep your spine aligned and your upper body supported.

Pillows come in a variety of styles, each offering different benefits. Some pillows are designed specifically to support the neck and back, while others benefit the whole body. You also want to consider your typical sleeping position when choosing your pillow because back sleepers, side sleepers, and stomach sleepers can each benefit from different styles of pillows.

The type of pillow you choose will depend on how much comfort and support you're seeking and whether you want a cloudlike pillow or a firmer pillow. It's helpful to talk to a professional, such as a chiropractor, to learn what type of pillow would be most suitable for you. Another option is to go to a mattress store and test various pillow styles to see what feels best for you.

A decent pillow is absolutely worth the investment for the kind of support and comfort required for restful quality sleep.

Use a Massage Gun

Releasing tension in your muscles is relaxing, and it's possible to do this activity regularly with a massage gun! Massage guns are an innovation to aid in the process of muscle recovery. They're small handheld devices that include various attachments to target many different areas of the body. Using a massage gun provides results similar to those from a deep tissue massage. They're great for increasing mobility, as they target your muscles, ligaments, tendons, and connective tissue.

Massage guns are easy to use on yourself, so you can feel comfortable while giving your body much-needed attention. Before you begin your massage, you will need to choose the type of attachment to use. You'll want to try all of them on different parts of your body to see which feels best. Massage guns come with instructions on the various attachments, so that can give you some guidance too. When turning on the device, start on the lowest setting and see how the vibrations feel. It can feel intense at first, but you will get used to it! Gradually increase the intensity and see what feels best to you.

You can find massage guns online ranging from $20 to several hundred dollars, so choose the style you find most appealing.

Practice Acupressure on Yourself

Acupressure is one of the most common methods of therapeutic treatment. It's a simple practice that involves pressing on acupoints and meridians with your fingers and hands. As a result of this therapy, both your mind and your body will feel relaxed and rejuvenated.

You can perform acupressure on yourself, making it possible to experience the countless benefits of this practice without going to a professional. However, it is imperative that you locate the correct pressure points on your body and are mindful to apply firm pressure on the various pressure points while using less pressure where you feel pain.

It is highly recommended that you read a book on acupressure or visit a trusted website to learn more about the different acupoints and meridians, as each point provides a distinct benefit and stimulates a different type of energy within the body. If you are trying to relieve pressure or tension in a particular area, make sure you know the correct acupoint for that pain point. Once you've identified the acupoints you'd like to target, use your finger pads to firmly hold pressure on that acupoint with a slight rotation or upward movement for at least two minutes. Practice daily for maximum benefit.

Play an Outdoor Game with a Friend

Participating in leisurely games and playing sports is beneficial for children and adults alike. Playing outdoor games with a friend is a great way to have fun, take life less seriously, and get your mind off responsibilities and daily duties.

Outdoor activities provide many of the same benefits as "green exercise," including exposure to vitamin D, fresh air, and psychological, physical, and social gains for all. A friendly competition also provides ample opportunity for bonding with your friend and deepening your connection.

The physical activity allows you to release any pent-up negative energy that's been building up within from the countless stressors you're faced with daily. Along with building self-confidence, you'll also feel happier, more relaxed, and a lot more carefree.

Call a friend on a day when the weather is nice and extend an invitation to join you for some fun in the sun! Find a local park with an open field or a basketball hoop—whatever you prefer—and choose a couple of activities that you and your friend are both familiar with and will both enjoy. Make sure to bring any required gear for the games you choose!

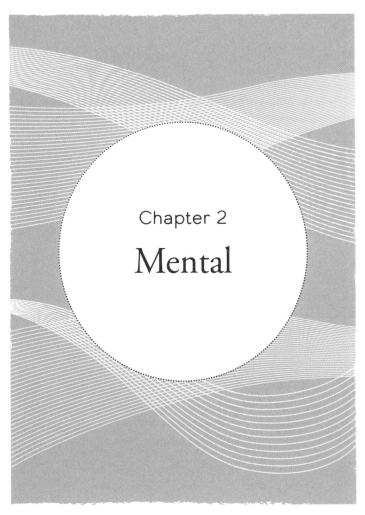

Chapter 2

Mental

Have you ever felt completely exhausted after a long day, but despite your physical fatigue, you can't fall asleep? That's because your body is at rest but your mind isn't.

Thousands of thoughts cross your mind each and every day. Whether you're conscious of it or not, thoughts are running through your mind incessantly in every waking moment. You are constantly inundated with a plethora of information and can feel overwhelmed by the enormous amount of content you consume daily. However, you can consciously choose to slow down, be mindful, and deliberately calm your mind and take a break from the senseless chatter. Allowing your mind to rest will provide you with a multitude of mental health benefits.

In this chapter you'll learn practical techniques to calm your mind anytime, anywhere. The activities range from listening to soothing music and meditating to playing board games and coloring. Many people find it uncomfortable to sit with their own thoughts or to be disconnected from their screens. The more you practice these activities, the easier it'll become.

Do a Ten-Minute
Relaxation Meditation

Relaxation meditation is one of the simplest and most beneficial ways to incorporate more rest and relaxation into your daily routine. Relaxation meditation provides many benefits including reduced stress, better mental and physical health, and more restful sleep. Meditation has a cumulative effect, so the longer you practice meditating on a consistent basis, the greater the impact it will have on your health. By practicing relaxation meditation for as little as ten minutes a day, you'll immediately feel more peaceful, calm, and relaxed.

1. Find a calm, quiet place and get comfortable.
2. Set a timer for ten minutes and close your eyes.
3. Bring your attention to your breath, following it as it goes in and out through your nose.
4. Begin counting your breaths (in-out one, in-out two, in-out three…) until you get to ten, and then start back at one. Continue this process until the timer goes off.
5. When you notice that your mind has wandered, don't judge yourself; just return your attention to your breath.
6. When your alarm goes off, slowly open your eyes and notice how good you feel!

Take a Thirty-Minute Break
from Your Phone

If you monitor your screen use, you just might notice that you spend more time on your electronic devices than you spend sleeping! It can be hard to take a break from your devices, especially when you rely on them for so many aspects of your life.

However, for you to experience mental rest and total relaxation, it is crucial for you to turn off your devices for at least thirty minutes each day, and this is highly recommended before bedtime.

Not only will turning off your devices relax your mind and promote better sleep, but limiting your screen time also reduces anxiety and eye strain. More importantly, when you put down your devices, you create more space for close relationships, mindfulness, and productivity.

Here are some tips to help you disconnect:

* Put your phone in "Do Not Disturb" mode. You can change the settings to receive phone calls only from specific contacts if you think they might need to reach you in case of an emergency.

* Create an automatic text message response informing the other person about your technology break and possible delay in response.
* Put your devices in another room so you are not tempted to check them.

Color in a Coloring Book

Coloring is a wonderful activity for practicing mindfulness and relaxation. Do you remember the carefree feeling of coloring as a child? You can still enjoy coloring! Adult coloring books are becoming increasingly popular, and the art of coloring has been found to significantly reduce stress and anxiety.

Coloring can be quite a meditative experience, which is why it's so relaxing. Like meditation, coloring has the ability to relax the amygdala, the fear center of the brain. Many of the designs filling the pages of adult coloring books include very intricate patterns, making the images extremely detailed and therefore requiring intense focus to color properly.

You might be thinking, "I don't have time to just sit and color!" but coloring doesn't require a lot of time. You can achieve the benefits of this activity in as little as ten minutes. To get started, visit your local bookstore, or browse the tens of thousands of adult coloring books available online, and pick the book that speaks to you the most. You will also need a set of colored pencils.

Anytime you are feeling a little stressed, pull out the coloring book and allow yourself to become immersed in the soothing process.

Declutter Your Closet

Decluttering your closet feels so rewarding! A clean, organized space also feels very relaxing. You can focus better when your living space is free of clutter. Too many things around you can be distracting to your mind and feel highly overwhelming.

As you begin going through each item, one by one, place each into one of four piles: keep, undecided, donate, or trash. Commit to throwing out any item that is stained, has a hole, or looks ratty for any reason, and immediately put it in the trash pile. Pull any items that you know you are keeping and place them in the keep pile.

Go through the items you felt undecided about and choose what to keep and what to donate. You should ask yourself the following questions for each item: "Have I worn it in the past year? Does it currently fit me? Do I love how this makes me feel?"

If you cannot answer yes to all three of these questions, donate it! If you do answer yes to all three, you should probably keep it!

Take all items you are donating to a shelter or donation box the same or very next day.

Start a Jigsaw Puzzle

An easy way to escape the chaos and commotion of everyday life is to complete a jigsaw puzzle. If you can't remember the last time you put together a colorful jigsaw puzzle, bring puzzles back into your life! You can spend some time doing this activity when you need a break from work or anytime you want to relax your racing mind.

Puzzles are an excellent exercise for working on your mental health as they require focused concentration on the task at hand, making it difficult to think about everything that's usually on your mind. As with traditional meditation, it is much easier to tune out the rest of the world when you focus on one thing. In addition to improving your focus and concentration, putting together a jigsaw puzzle eases stress and anxiety as the racing, anxious thoughts begin to subside.

Choosing a puzzle that speaks to you will make completing a jigsaw puzzle even more fun. Clear up some space, perhaps on a large table, so you can easily spread out the puzzle pieces. Turn on some relaxing music and enjoy getting lost in the puzzle and escaping reality for just a little bit.

Read a Fiction Book

One simple way to relax your mind is to read a good fiction book. Besides being a fun hobby, reading fictional stories also has several health benefits. If you can devote even thirty minutes a day to reading for enjoyment, you could start to experience lower heart rate, blood pressure, and anxiety levels.

In addition to the physical benefits, just sitting down to read a book can positively change your mindset as well, as this genre is usually entertaining, fun, and relaxing. These things are all important for your mental health because they allow your mind to rest and detach from the concerns of everyday life. Reading an exciting novel can be a fun escape, especially if you're hooked on the book. Reading before bed is also a great way to unwind and relax your mind, and can help you fall asleep faster.

If you really want to use your reading time to escape the real world, designate a space in your home for reading and limit distractions to the best of your ability. You can add a comfortable chair or beanbag, a relaxing light, comfortable pillows, and a soft blanket. Enjoy your book and the pure relaxation that comes with it!

Walk Outside While Listening to an Audiobook

Who said you can't multitask and experience relaxation at the same time? Taking a leisurely walk around the neighborhood while listening to an audiobook you enjoy can be a truly relaxing experience. If you combine low-impact physical exercise with a low-impact mental activity like active listening, you benefit mentally as well as physically. For anyone who finds walking around the neighborhood boring, this is the perfect activity.

Your mood and attitude can be positively impacted by listening to audiobooks. If you suffer from anxiety or depression, listening to someone else read can relieve your stress by making you focus on something specific instead of negative thoughts. Along with relaxing your mind, you will also relax your eyes since you won't have to read in a book or look at a screen.

The easiest way to listen to an audiobook while walking outside is to download an audiobook app on your phone. Many paid apps are available, but you can usually find free options through your local library's audiobook app. Browse through whatever genres interest you and choose a book you think you'll enjoy! Remember to wear headphones so you can fully enjoy your new book!

Soak in a Hot Tub

Soaking in a hot tub at the end of a long day or stressful week can be a wonderful way to unwind and is extremely relaxing for your body and mind. Hot tubs are a pleasant reminder of what it feels like to relax on vacation. Just imagine the hot water melting your worries away and helping you escape the stress of the day. Hot tubs are often known for relaxing the mind, but it turns out that spending time in a hot tub may offer even more health benefits. The jets in the hot tub can relieve stiff and tense muscles, reduce pain, and help prevent injury. Your mind and body will feel so relaxed afterward that you may even end up getting a better night's sleep.

If you don't have a hot tub at your home, many spas and fitness centers have hot tubs you can use. Check that the hot tub is set at a temperature below 103°F before getting in. Water that is too hot can cause discomfort and even light-headedness. Spend no more than fifteen to twenty minutes in the hot tub; relax your racing mind and let it reach its Zen state. Remember to also stay hydrated during your spa session and focus on your breathing.

Practice Deep Breathing

Breathing is a vital part of our existence, yet it often gets ignored. Your breath is one of the most powerful tools available to help you cope with everyday stress and feel calmer and more relaxed in any moment.

The pace and depth of your breath is an indicator of the level of stress you may be experiencing. Shallow breaths are a sign that your nervous system is heightened in anxiety. Deep breaths that make your belly expand are what you should strive for. There are countless benefits to deep breathing, including lower blood pressure, less anxiety, increased energy, improved digestion, and enhanced focus. Try the following deep-breathing practice:

1. Find a comfortable place to sit or lie down.
2. Close your eyes.
3. Place one hand on your heart and the other on your belly.
4. Notice the current state of your breath. Is it shallow? Is it steady?
5. Take a long inhale through your nose, aiming for a count of four.

6. Hold your breath at the top of the inhale for a count of four.
7. Slowly and fully exhale the air through your nose for a count of four.
8. Repeat these steps for about five minutes.

Visualize a Stress-Free Day

Visualization is a simple and powerful practice that anyone can do. When you practice visualization, you are envisioning what you want your future self to experience and feel. In this activity, you will specifically visualize less stress, so you can attract more rest. When you visualize a day free from stress, you will begin to feel calmer and more relaxed about what lies in front of you for the day. Try this technique in the morning to get yourself off on the right foot for a calm and relaxing day. Depending on your comfort level, you can meditate for anywhere between five and thirty minutes. Here's how to do it.

Close your eyes and take a few long, deep breaths. Once you've settled into a relaxed state, you can begin the visualization exercise. The most important aspect of a visualization practice is to fully experience the desired feelings. The best way to do this is by utilizing as many senses as possible. For example, your idea of a stress-free day could be a fun, playful, and relaxing day at the beach. So for your visualization practice, you will want to envision yourself at the beach on a beautiful, sunny day. You want to be very detailed in your mind, imagining the sound of the waves crashing on the shore, the smell of the salt water in the air, the feeling of the sand beneath your feet, the warm sun on your face, and so on. Most importantly, you want to try to *feel* the desired feelings of being stress-free, carefree, relaxed, playful, and joyful, and really focus on those feelings as if you were experiencing them in this moment.

Ask for Help with Household Chores

Household chores can be extremely overwhelming and the antithesis of relaxation and rest. That's why it's important to remember that asking for help with them is okay! Create a weekly cleaning schedule for every family member. Organize the daily tasks in a way that makes them manageable for everyone. A little bit will get done each day, and by the end of the week, all the chores will be complete! If it isn't possible to ask household members for assistance, you can also think about hiring a cleaning company. This can be a practical option for busy people and can help relieve a lot of stress.

By allowing someone else to take care of all or a part of the weekly cleaning for you, you can take time for yourself and your family. Don't feel bad about asking for help or hiring someone to help you. Your mental wellness is essential, and relieving yourself of additional responsibilities can be extremely beneficial to you and your family in the long run.

Remember, you can't pour from an empty cup, and you shouldn't have to be responsible for managing everything in your home. Put together a schedule for your family or contact a local cleaning service so you can make some space in your life for doing things that bring you joy and relaxation.

Consume Less News

The news tends to bombard us with one tragedy after another, which takes a massive toll on our mental health and well-being. The constant consumption of negativity, fear, and worldwide suffering can leave you feeling as though the world is a horrible place and the future for humanity is hopeless.

We've been programmed to believe it's necessary for us to stay informed on what is going on all over the world, but this isn't necessarily true. Constantly consuming the news by watching TV, reading articles online or in newspapers, listening to the radio, and so on can do more harm than good.

Simply detaching yourself from this endless barrage will do wonders for your mental health! Although you may feel anxious and uncomfortable initially from feeling like you're not staying informed, you will quickly realize how much more peaceful and relaxed you feel in general! You will also have so much more space in your mind to focus on what's important to you.

Remove all news apps from your devices, unsubscribe from any media and news outlets, and inform your family and friends that you no longer wish to discuss anything news related, or negative for that matter! You will discover you will find a new sense of calm and focus once you turn off the news.

Go on a Camping Trip

Camping is a wonderful way to rest, relax, and regroup. Your physical environment can significantly affect your ability to rest and relax. In a world where you are constantly on the go, it can be hard to clear your mind when you return home, especially if you associate your home with stress. Taking a break from your usual routine and surroundings and spending time in nature are both excellent ways to improve your mental health.

In addition, camping trips usually consist of a variety of relaxing activities such as walking in nature, hiking, meditating, building a campfire, lying in a hammock, and taking naps. Just the feeling of being so far away from all your usual responsibilities and daily stressors can be soothing.

Ask your partner or a couple of friends to go on a fun-filled yet relaxing adventure with you! Then decide if you want to rent a cabin or an RV or go au naturel and camp in a tent. This decision will help you figure out the type of campsite to book. Once you've found the perfect camping spot, call the campground or visit their website and book your stay. Then relax and have some fun!

Take the Weekend Off from the Internet

The Internet is an unavoidable part of our lives, and it can serve many positive purposes. Nevertheless, it is easy to become completely addicted to and dependent on the Internet, whether for work or entertainment. This constant need to check, scroll, and post takes a toll on your inner calm and can make it hard to slow down and relax. In addition, it's been proven that social media sites can promote depression and negative feelings about yourself—neither of which is very relaxing!

It's common in today's world to feel like you always need to be available to others and respond immediately to text messages and emails. But why should you? The constant stimuli from technology can be very draining. Instead, try making an effort to completely unplug from the Internet at least one weekend every month. Yes, this means no Internet usage on your phone or laptop. No emails either! All you need to do is shut down your computer and other devices that you use to access the Internet. If you want to avoid feeling tempted to use your phone, ask your family to hold you accountable for your Internet-free weekend. Tell them you will check your phone only for important calls or messages three times a day. Your family will love this present version of you!

You might notice that you're more focused and experience better sleep without the distraction of the Internet. Being present in your weekend activities will be easier too!

Practice Mindfulness During Meals

Do you pay attention to your food while eating or do you eat mindlessly? Maybe it's time to try some mindful eating during your meals!

Mindful eating simply involves paying attention to your food without judging the food or yourself. It creates a calm and peaceful experience around eating and can make your meals feel more relaxed and enjoyable. This isn't about paying attention to the nutritional value of the food you are eating, but instead to how it tastes, smells, and makes you feel. Cultivate an awareness of the experience you receive when eating a particular food. Your meals will be more enjoyable if you can savor the moment and be fully present. You will also feel more grateful for your food if you can enjoy it in this way.

By practicing mindful eating, you will be present during mealtime and develop better eating habits. You can choose one meal a day to dedicate to mindfulness. Make sure you don't bring any distractions to the table, like cell phones or magazines. Chew your food slowly, and don't rush your meal. Paying attention to each bite you take during meals can reduce binge eating, help you lose weight, and promote better digestion. Although it may seem strange at first, you will enjoy the benefits that come from this activity!

Plan a Vacation

The act of planning a vacation can bring joy, excitement, and peace to your mind. Knowing that you will soon be able to unwind from the daily grind in a beautiful, peaceful environment you have chosen for yourself is a comforting thought. Visiting a new spot can be the perfect way to break away from your daily routine and give your mind some much-needed rest.

First, decide whether you want to take a solo trip or invite friends or family. If you are bringing friends and family along, it can be fun to plan the details together!

Once you have figured out who is going and where you are going to vacation, the real fun begins in choosing all the details! Enjoy the process of choosing a place to stay, activities you will do, and sights you want to explore! Sometimes, planning your vacation can be just as fun as the actual trip.

The planning process is like practicing visualization because you automatically begin to envision yourself on the vacation experiencing each of the activities you are choosing for your trip. Enjoying your mental vacation before your actual vacation can be a great mood boost and can help you feel more positive and calm about your day.

Watch Funny Animal Videos

There's just something so satisfying about watching adorable, funny animal videos! If you want to relax or have a good laugh while killing time, this can be a great way to do it. There's so much to explore, from cat and dog videos to footage of animals in the wild. The simple act of watching videos of cute animals can calm your mind and help you decompress. Browse animal accounts on your favorite social media platforms. Find the accounts that speak the most to you, and take five minutes to see what they have recently posted. Often when people use social media, they tend to inadvertently come across negative news, so deliberately choosing to follow positive, funny, and uplifting accounts that bring you peace can make you feel more at ease.

If you use social media daily, you can make watching animal videos part of your routine. Since you have found the accounts that share positive and funny videos, you can take five minutes each day and visit their accounts before continuing your social media scroll. This can make your online experience more fun and lighter, which is a great way to escape the chaos for a few minutes.

Listen to a Motivational Podcast

Need more inspiration and/or motivation in your life? Listen to podcasts! Download a free podcast app on your phone for daily inspiration. These audio shows vary from educational to entertaining and everything in between. There are so many enlightening podcasts to choose from, many of which can completely transform your outlook on life!

Many people try to multitask while listening to podcasts; however, it can be more relaxing to mindfully listen to a podcast when you are driving, walking, or taking some time to rest. To rest while listening, lie down somewhere comfortable, close your eyes, and let the positive audio flow through your ears. Have a notebook nearby in case you want to write down anything that comes to mind. Focus on the words you are hearing so you can fully absorb the information. As you notice that your mind is wandering and you are thinking about things unrelated to the audio, just gently guide your focus back to the audio and rewind it a minute or two in case you missed something essential.

Taking the time to listen to motivational information is a wonderful way to learn, grow, and evolve, while simultaneously allowing your body and mind to rest.

Order a Healthy Meal "To Go"

Cooking a meal at home after a long day at work might just be the last thing you feel like doing, but you might very well feel obligated to! Thinking about having to go through the rigors of cooking can sometimes feel anything but relaxing. Instead, treat yourself to delivery or carryout and save yourself the stress of shopping, preparation, cooking, and cleaning up! There are plenty of restaurants that make healthy, nutritious, and delicious meals. Figure out what you're in the mood to eat and pick a healthy option from the menu. Then use your newfound free time to sit back and relax and do something that brings you joy.

At least once a week, try to treat yourself and indulge in a healthy take-out meal. Give yourself this occasional but much-needed break from the never-ending list of things you are responsible for every day. If you're adamant that once a week is not possible with your budget, at least try to make this a priority once or twice a month. It will be worth the investment for the time and stress it saves you.

To make this even more fun and exciting, choose an intriguing new tasty dish each week!

Play a Board Game

Playing board games can be an excellent way to clear your mind and relax. As an added bonus, board games are often nostalgic, bringing back memories and feelings of playing games when you were a child. Plus, playing more board games equals less screen time so it's a win-win!

Get your family and friends together and play a game that everyone can enjoy. To experience the benefits of playing a board game, ensure that all members are committed to playing the game without disturbances. Remove all electronic devices from the room you will be playing in and be present in the moment. This allows everyone to relax and turn their minds from the distractions of everyday life by focusing all their attention on a little friendly competition!

If you plan to host a game night with friends and family, set up your game space in a room that's full of positive energy. Prepare the space for a good time by adding snacks and beverages for the players and turning on music that everyone will enjoy. Have two to three different games and vote to choose between them.

Playing a simple board game provides a lot of fun and an opportunity for stress reduction and connection with others.

Journal Your Thoughts

Journaling is an effective way to relax your mind. When you write in a journal, you take all the incessant thoughts constantly overwhelming your mind and put them down on paper. This simple activity is extremely powerful and can feel very therapeutic, like a weight is being released.

Journaling does not need to feel like a formal activity. Make it a habit to simply sit down and be still for a few minutes without distractions and just write. Let your thoughts and feelings flow freely and just witness them—write them down with no judgment, just awareness. Many people like to do this first thing in the morning or right before they go to bed at night. Anytime you're feeling stressed out or uneasy, allow yourself the freedom to just express it and let it out.

If you aren't used to journaling, this activity may feel weird at first, but you'll soon find that it can bring you comfort and peace. By keeping a journal, you allow your thoughts to escape your mind onto the paper instead of letting them consume you.

If you sit to write in your journal and nothing begins to flow, there are thousands of free journaling prompts online that can help you get your thoughts going.

Diffuse Essential Oils

An essential oil is a concentrated plant extract. Smelling these oils is thought to reduce stress and help restore emotional balance. You can experience an essential oil by using a diffuser, which allows the oil to evaporate and spread its scent throughout your home.

It's important to buy 100 percent pure oils from a reputable company. Some popular essential oils are:

* **EUCALYPTUS:** This scent calms the mind and can serve as a decongestant.
* **PEPPERMINT:** Peppermint is a popular oil to diffuse in an office while working or studying. It's helpful for headaches and can help clear your sinuses. It's perfect for a mental break.
* **LAVENDER:** This is the perfect oil to diffuse before bed. It helps calm the nervous system and helps prepare your mind for sleep.
* **ORANGE:** This oil can help reduce your stress levels and ease digestion issues.

You can find essential oils and oil diffusers in many stores and online. You will want to follow the instructions provided for your specific diffuser regarding the amount of water and number of drops of oil to use.

Turn Off Unnecessary Notifications

If you keep track of your screen time and data usage, you're obviously aware of how much time you spend using your phone each day. But what you may not be aware of is the negative impact the numerous apps and countless notifications have on your sense of calm and your mental state every time you swipe open your phone.

For example, you could be swiping open your phone to listen to a podcast—a relaxing and enjoyable activity. But before you even open the podcast app, your eyes notice the numerous notification bubbles spanning the screen, alerting you of unread emails, unopened Snapchat snaps or stories, or unwatched *YouTube* videos—and while you may not care about any of those things, your brain doesn't know that! The very second your eyes register the colorful bubbles, your brain immediately begins trying to process all the information. Your brain knows what each of those notifications is telling you based on experience, and therefore your mind instantaneously feels overwhelmed with information overload, which then causes you to feel anxious and stressed as an automatic response.

In order to avoid this wave of anxiety, turn off any unnecessary notifications so when you do use your phone or device you won't be putting your mental health in jeopardy. By turning off your notifications, you can help ensure a more peaceful and restful day.

Open a Savings Account

Many people in our society live paycheck to paycheck and have accrued substantial amounts of debt, making it nearly impossible to ever get ahead. Understandably, financial concerns are some of the greatest sources of stress and anxiety for most people.

One simple way to ease some of your stressful financial concerns is to open a savings account. Even if you live paycheck to paycheck and don't believe you make enough money to save any, just try it! If you receive direct deposits from your employer, you can allocate a percentage of the overall paycheck amount or a specific dollar amount to be directly deposited into your savings account each pay period. Even if you start with just 5 percent or $50 each pay period, you will notice a sense of pride and accomplishment in watching it accrue over time. Setting up your savings through direct deposit is especially nice because you never have the money in your hands, and you don't have to think about it.

It's comforting to contribute to your savings account monthly, knowing you're doing something positive for your financial well-being.

Practice Guided Imagery

A highly effective yet easy technique for relaxing the mind is guided imagery. Guided imagery is different from visual meditation in that it does not focus on your future desires and feelings, but on using scenic imagery in meditation to relax. Your brain cannot tell the difference between your experiencing an event in real life and your imagining that you are experiencing an event in your mind. Therefore, imagining that you are having positive experiences can be just as beneficial as actually experiencing them.

Guided imagery does not require any special tools. All you need are your imagination and a quiet, comfortable space. You can find guided imagery videos on *YouTube* that may be helpful when you are new to this practice. It can be helpful to follow along with their instructions and go through the process step-by-step.

To begin your practice, sit comfortably or lie down as you would when meditating. Close your eyes, softening your facial muscles, and take a few slow, deep breaths. Focus on your breathing. Now begin thinking about a place that brings you peace, such as a garden, beach, or forest. Imagine yourself there now. How does it feel? What can you hear? Who is with you? Spend about fifteen minutes in your happy place letting your imagination run free.

Limit Your TV Time

Watching TV can be mentally taxing. Most people think of watching TV as a passive, relaxing activity, but this isn't necessarily the case. Many studies have found that our brains are anything but inactive when we watch TV. Not to mention that watching TV tends to consume a massive amount of time and energy—time and energy that we could be using to do things that bring us joy and fulfillment.

Instead of watching TV, spend your newfound free time reading books on topics you are passionate about, listening to enlightening podcasts, spending quality time connecting with your loved ones, and sleeping.

Making the transition from being someone who watches several hours of TV daily to becoming someone who rarely watches TV can be challenging initially. However, if you commit to this practice and limit your TV time, you will be pleasantly surprised at the countless positive changes you experience as a result. Your overall health and well-being will improve immensely from making this one simple change. Notice, this doesn't say *easy*, but rather *simple*.

Try designating daily times for watching TV and committing to them—for example, 7:00 p.m.–8:00 p.m. on weeknights and 8:00 p.m.–10:00 p.m. on weekends.

Limit Your Work Time

These days, many people work from home full-time. This often comes with an expectation of always being plugged in and available when others may need us, and this can feel a bit overwhelming at times.

Having to be always "on call" for work can be stressful and anxiety-inducing, and cause you to have a negative outlook on life. It is important that you take breaks from working to avoid this type of burnout. To work effectively and efficiently, you must take time to rest and recharge. Working too much can negatively impact your sleep, physical and mental health, relationships, and so on.

Here are some tips:

* Throughout your workday, for every hour you spend working, take a five-minute break. Use this time to stand up, stretch, hydrate, and so on.
* Establish a time at which you will stop working each day and commit to it. Set an alarm to go off fifteen minutes prior to that time.
* Begin each day with a list of the three most important things you need to accomplish that day, and do them in order of importance or deadline.
* Avoid multitasking. Concentrate on completing one task at a time, little by little.

Take the Day Off

When you work for an employer, there is a reason they offer vacation time and sick leave. Mental rest days are critical for your mental health. Even if you don't work for someone else, it is necessary to give yourself a day off from your normal responsibilities occasionally.

If you have been feeling particularly burned out, take a day off to do nothing but rest. Choose a few activities from this book that you'd like to complete on your mental rest day to ensure you are making the best use of this time you have given yourself to rest and relax.

If you really want to treat yourself, you can spend the day at the beach or spa. Fill your day with things that make you happy and leave you feeling refreshed. You will notice how much better you feel mentally after you've taken some time off from work. This is important for your health, so prioritize days off and start adding them to your schedule. Create a list of things you want to do to rejuvenate and reenergize your mind. No matter what, don't feel guilty for taking the day off! You deserve time to rest.

Delegate Your To-Do List

It's unrealistic to expect that you can handle all the tasks and responsibilities in your life entirely on your own. And even if you could, it doesn't mean you should. Trying to do everything yourself will eventually lead you to feel overwhelmed, stressed, and burned out.

It's time to delegate some of your tasks to others and create more balance in your life so you can rest more. To determine what tasks to delegate, ask yourself:

* Which tasks are repetitive and time-consuming?
* Is there anything I would be happier if I did not have to do?
* What tasks are easy for someone else to do?
* Are there essential tasks that I should let a professional handle?

To determine what you *shouldn't* delegate, ask yourself:

* What are some of the things I am good at and enjoy doing?
* What are things that only I can complete?
* Are there any confidential tasks that only I should be handling?

If you're unsure about delegating, ask yourself why. Does this stem from a fear of losing control? If so, this is an excellent opportunity to dig deeper and explore this fear so you can work on overcoming it. The help of someone else can go a long way toward creating more balance in your life.

Complete a Project That's Been Causing You Stress

Although the action required to complete a stressful project is not a restful or relaxing activity, the resulting relief and inner peace you will feel are totally worth it! You will be able to relax more and rest easier once the project is no longer weighing on your mind.

Do you have any item on your to-do list that you constantly put off and never feel like doing, even though it's necessary? Do you feel stressed and anxious as a result? Do you notice it weighing on your mind when you are trying to fall asleep or at any other time? Then completing the project is the best solution! It feels so rewarding to cross an item off your to-do list, no matter how big or small.

If the project you are contemplating feels daunting because it's large or time-consuming, another option is breaking it down into smaller, more manageable tasks. Each time you complete one of those, you will feel proud and gain momentum to move on to another task! Either way, whether you complete the project or break it down and begin completing parts of the project, this will give you more headspace and allow you to rest.

Try Release Writing

Release writing is a powerful tool that can give you much-needed relief and help you relax and rest. Release writing is a fast-paced "stream of consciousness" process used to dump your thoughts and feelings while writing by hand.

Most people tend to avoid their feelings because they fear them or because it's what they've been taught to do. However, avoiding and suppressing your feelings is extremely draining on your energy, and the long-term impact of this is far greater than the short-term pain you would experience by processing them. When you suppress your negative feelings, you are storing negative energy in your body. Unexpressed sadness typically causes lethargy and depression, and unexpressed anger often manifests as anxiety and irritability.

Release writing is a simple activity that you can try in order to release these negative emotions. You simply write as fast as you can while keeping up with your thoughts as best as you can. Do not analyze, judge, interpret, or go back and reread what you wrote. Just write and release!

To give it a try, begin by writing, "I feel sad because," or, "I feel angry because," and then keep writing! Really allow yourself to feel the feelings as you write, and don't stop until you experience a sense of emptiness and relief. Upon completion, safely destroy the paper to release the energy entirely.

Sit Around a Campfire

Spending time outside and in nature can be incredibly relaxing, allowing you to let go of stress and tension.

While you are sitting around a campfire, there are so many relaxing activities to choose from:

* Socialize with friends or family without the presence of technology.
* Read a book that brings you joy.
* Make food over the fire and/or roast marshmallows.
* Close your eyes and meditate while focusing on the warmth on your skin.
* Let your creativity flow and write in your journal.
* Watch animals play nearby.
* Watch the sunrise or sunset.
* Listen to peaceful music or play your own instrument.
* Sit in stillness and savor the peaceful ambience.

Regardless of what you choose to do while sitting around a campfire, you will benefit from the peacefulness and tranquility the fire elicits. Sitting outside in the cool air while simultaneously feeling the warmth radiating from the fire is very soothing. The next time you are looking to take a break from your routine and enjoy simple, relaxing activities on your own or with others, make a campfire!

Listen to Binaural Beats

We all know that music can positively impact our energy and mood, but did you know that just listening to sounds can do this also? Specifically, listening to binaural beats.

When you hear two different tones, one in each ear, with slightly different frequencies, your brain processes a beat that is the difference between the two frequencies, and this is referred to as a binaural beat. Binaural beats are considered auditory illusions.

Binaural beats between 1 Hz and 30 Hz tend to create brain wave patterns similar to those experienced during meditation. Listening to binaural beats can help relieve tension, encourage creativity, enhance feelings of happiness, decrease anxiety, improve focus and concentration, and increase relaxation. Listening to binaural beats should be done in a quiet, comfortable space, free of distractions. You must use headphones so that each ear is hearing the different frequencies.

If you want to explore the benefits of binaural beats, you just need a binaural beat sound source and headphones. You can search "binaural beats for relaxation" on *YouTube* and find an abundant selection to choose from. Listen to several options to find the beats that resonate with you the most and make you feel the most peaceful and relaxed.

Reduce Your Caffeine Intake

Have you felt particularly restless or anxious lately? Your caffeine intake may be the culprit. This stimulant appears in coffee and tea, as well as in other foods and beverages. Our tendency to turn to caffeinated beverages is not only because of their desirable taste but also because they give us a perceived burst of energy shortly after we drink them.

However, consuming too much caffeine can also have negative effects, such as causing you to feel jittery, increasing your anxiety and stress, raising your blood pressure, increasing headaches and stomachaches, and inducing insomnia.

Drinking too much caffeine can disturb your sleep patterns, causing you to experience restless sleep at night and to feel sleepy during the day. This then makes you feel like you need to drink more caffeine throughout the day, and the cycle continues.

Try avoiding caffeine after breakfast. If you like having caffeine throughout the day, consider having a cutoff time to stop consuming caffeine to help you sleep better at night. Commit to avoiding caffeine at least six hours before going to bed.

Don't worry, you can still enjoy your favorite coffee or tea! But limiting your daily consumption of caffeine will help you achieve better quality sleep and rest.

Eliminate or Limit Alcohol

If you're striving for optimal health, it's in your best interest to eliminate alcohol entirely, or at the very least, significantly limit your alcohol intake. While some studies show modest cardiovascular benefits associated with moderate drinking, that small effect is overshadowed by the numerous ways alcohol can threaten your health. People who drink alcohol increase their risk of obesity, diabetes, cancer, cirrhosis of the liver, kidney failure, heart diseases, mental health issues, injuries, and traffic accidents.

Alcohol also negatively affects your sleep. Many people drink alcohol to "unwind and relax" and have convinced themselves that drinking alcohol before bed helps them sleep. The reality is, alcohol prevents you from entering a deep sleep cycle, which is necessary to restore and heal your body. When you quit drinking, you'll be amazed at how much better you sleep, and, consequently, how much better you feel overall.

In the alcohol-centric world we live in, it might seem impossible to quit your alcohol consumption, but an alcohol-free existence offers many benefits that are ultimately more rewarding than a temporary buzz. Once you learn how to live without this toxic crutch, your life will be more restful and peaceful.

Learn to Say No

We often find it difficult to say no to others' requests, especially when they want us to attend an event or need our help. We are used to saying yes to everything because we feel the weight of people's expectations of us and have been taught to put others first.

However, living this way is exhausting, is overwhelming, and leads to burnout because your schedule is always packed, and it leaves you no time for yourself, and no time to rest or replenish your own energy.

When you say no to things you don't want to do, it makes you feel empowered and in control, frees up your time, allows more time for rest, and makes you stronger mentally. Contrary to our societal programming, self-preservation should be your number one priority, not other people's expectations. This is a much healthier way to live!

The next time someone asks you to do something, pause and take the time to ask yourself: Do I really want to do this? Am I just people-pleasing? Is this going to add to my well-being or subtract from it? Then feel empowered to politely say no if you don't want to do the activity. Only you can protect your own peace!

Listen to Classical Music

Listening to classical music offers countless mental and physical benefits. Listening to classical music (even just as background noise) increases your happiness, boosts your mood, sparks creativity, supercharges your brainpower, improves memory, increases productivity, decreases blood pressure, relieves pain, fights depression, reduces anxiety and stress levels, and helps you fall asleep faster and achieve better quality sleep.

The brain responds well to classical music because the tempo is usually slower and the gentle sounds of string instruments are soothing. Instead of watching TV before bed, try listening to classical music for the last forty-five minutes to an hour before your bedtime and see if it improves your sleep and how you feel throughout the following day! You'll likely feel better rested and more relaxed.

This genre of music is the perfect choice to listen to if you are looking to create a peaceful, relaxing, and joyful environment in your home, at work, while working out, before bed, or anytime! There are many outstanding classical music artists, but to start, you can consider listening to some pieces by Johann Sebastian Bach, Ludwig van Beethoven, Frédéric Chopin, Claude Debussy, and Wolfgang Amadeus Mozart.

Practice Better Time Management Skills

Would you like to have more time to rest and spend less time worrying about your to-do list? We all have the same twenty-four hours in a day; the only difference is the way we spend them! Learning better time management skills and practices helps you accomplish more in less time and decreases the amount of stress and anxiety you experience.

When you create a system of accomplishing things efficiently, you will feel so much more relaxed mentally. It isn't about getting all your tasks done in one day, but it is about creating a plan to have sufficient time to complete what's most important to you. With better time management, you will accomplish all that truly needs to be done and have more time to rest and unwind.

Start by writing down your entire to-do list. Then, prioritize your tasks by asking yourself what is most urgent and essential. Schedule those tasks to be completed early in the day and in the week. Getting the biggest, most important jobs out of the way first will help you feel better mentally, reduce the amount of time you stress over getting them done, and allow you more time to relax when you are finished.

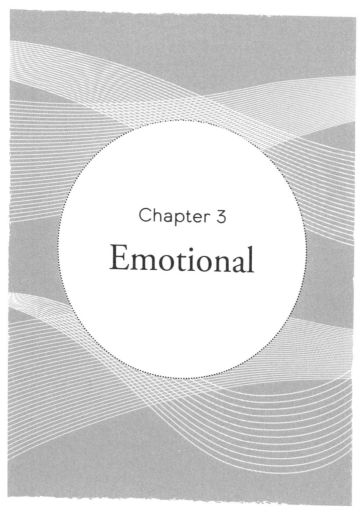

Chapter 3

Emotional

Are you ready to feel better and more rejuvenated? This chapter will help you accomplish that! When you are in touch with your feelings, you will start to realize which thoughts and actions bring more positivity to your life. Take note of how you feel before and after the activities in this chapter. Your emotions may differ each time, but be sure to keep coming back to the activities that bring out the most restful and relaxing feelings.

Prioritizing your emotional well-being is part of emotional rest. Many of the activities in this chapter promote emotional well-being, such as spending time daydreaming, doing laughter yoga, watching funny movies, and practicing gratitude. To experience emotional rest, you also need to find ways to reduce stress. Many of the activities in this chapter help you reduce stress, such as having difficult conversations you've been avoiding, allowing yourself to cry, and releasing judgment. You will love how much better you feel and how much more rest you experience as a result of getting in touch with, accepting, and releasing your emotions.

Cuddle with a Pet

There's a reason people like to cuddle with their cat or dog when they're feeling anxious or stressed out. Pets have a seemingly magical calming effect on humans. Whether it's a dog, cat, rabbit, or hamster, cuddling with a pet can make you feel supported, calm, and comforted. Pets have a way of giving humans unconditional love, support, attention, and acceptance that is unmatched by anything else.

Studies have shown that petting or hugging a loving animal can rapidly calm and soothe you when you're stressed or anxious. Spending time with a pet has also been shown to ease loneliness, decrease depression, and reduce blood pressure in stressful situations.

Here are some tips for making the most out of your snuggle sesh:

* Petting animals has been shown to reduce the stress hormone cortisol, so don't hesitate to gently stroke their back and head or rub their tummy.
* Try to be present in the moment by noticing how their fur feels, their mannerisms, or any sounds they make.
* You can also look into your pet's eyes. Mutual eye gaze enhances the human-animal bond and has positive effects on human health and well-being.

Appreciate Small Moments of Joy

Do you appreciate the little things in life? Have you heard the saying "When you focus on the good, the good gets better"? It's so true! When you deliberately take notice of all the wonderful things around you, you suddenly become aware of more and more amazing things to appreciate. When you notice this good, it will improve your mood, which in turn will reduce your stress and anxiety about life and allow you to feel more calm and relaxed.

Most people are unconsciously going through life in default mode, rushing from one thing to the next, always busy and distracted, and completely oblivious to the magic happening all around them. Being present and mindful is a much more relaxing way to live than most of us are used to.

Some ways to appreciate the small moments in life every day are:

* Wake up twenty minutes earlier than usual so you can experience your morning routine without rushing.
* Savor the flavors in every bite of food or every sip of coffee, and so on.
* Sit outside and observe the sunrise or sunset, and bask in the exquisite beauty of the ombré sky.

Don't wait for life to be easy, as it will always be complex. Situations can't always be controlled, but how you experience them can be. Choose to slow down and focus on things that make you happy every day.

Spend Ten Minutes Daydreaming

Daydreaming isn't just a fun way to escape reality; it's also a healthy habit for relaxation, since your mind cannot constantly maintain focus and productivity. In terms of mental well-being, daydreaming works similarly to meditation as it allows you to rest your mind in a healthy way. By tuning out the "outside" world, you can free up your thoughts.

Daydreaming involves allowing your mind to wander as you create fantasies with your imagination. The fun thing about daydreaming is that there are no rules! You can allow yourself to dream about anything you want—just make sure it is positive. This will ensure that the experience is both relaxing and enjoyable!

Daydreaming isn't really a practice to just sit down and do. Studies have found that this is difficult for most people. Rather, you want to allow this practice to happen naturally. If at any time you become aware of the fact that you are daydreaming, just allow your mind to wander. If you notice it wandering when you are working, it might be telling you it needs a break. So, allow yourself to daydream for about ten minutes. Daydreaming is beneficial to your emotional health and leads to more creative ideas.

Visit a Botanical Garden

Visiting a local botanical garden can be a relaxing and joyful activity. Taking time to appreciate the beauty of nature can give you a sense of peace and lift your spirits, and may even decrease anxiety.

Research local botanical gardens or look for one that you're willing to take a trip to. Botanical gardens make wonderful day trips! Many gardens are open to the public year-round, so you can make this a regular outing by yourself or with a friend.

Pack plenty of water and snacks or maybe even a picnic lunch if there isn't a place to buy food in the gardens. Wear sunscreen and comfortable clothing and walking shoes so you can move freely throughout the day.

Botanical gardens typically have long walking paths, so your body can benefit from the light activity as you relax your mind at the same time. Practice mindfulness and stay present in the moment during your visit. You can also practice gratitude for the wonders of nature and your ability to enjoy them. Explore as much as you can and take in all the sights as you go. You might even feel inspired to re-create some of the displays in your own backyard!

Reconnect with a Friend

Reconnecting with a good friend can help you feel loved and supported. Our lives can feel overwhelming with never-ending to-do lists, but it's important to schedule time for socializing and relaxing with friends.

Whether you get together in person or just reconnect over the phone, be present during your time together. Catching up on what you have both been up to and any positive changes that have occurred in either of your lives can be fun and exciting. On the other hand, if any negative changes have occurred, the other person may really need a friend right now to be there for them, and you may have felt called to reach out just when they needed someone the most, to offer them love, compassion, and support. Feelings of connectedness with others are conducive to emotional well-being and can feel very fulfilling.

There are various ways to stay connected with friends, even if you live far away or can't meet up in person. You can simply give them a call, video chat, send them an email or a text message, or even send them a card or handwritten note just to let them know you are thinking of them.

Watch a Positive TV Show

Did you know that the shows you watch on TV greatly influence your emotional well-being? So many people watch TV to "relax" and are completely unaware that the shows they are watching are causing them serious distress. This is because most people have very little self-awareness.

How have you been feeling during TV time recently? If you have been consuming shows that make you feel anxious or upset in any way, it might be time to change up your nightly lineup! It can be hard to determine how a show will make you feel before starting to watch it, so if you feel any discomfort, or notice feeling tension in your body within the first thirty minutes of watching, then it is time to try another show.

If you have noticed that any genres make you feel negative, stay away from them. Narrowing down your options to genres that make you feel good can make TV show exploration more successful. There are no benefits to watching anxiety-inducing TV. If someone else in your household is watching something that doesn't feel good to you, leave the room! It's up to you to protect your own peace!

Listen to Ocean Waves

A trip to the beach is never complete without hearing the waves crashing against the shore! We often feel peaceful when we're at the beach because listening to the waves is relaxing to our mind. The ease and flow of the water's constant movement is soothing, meditative, and calming to both watch and listen to. This is also a wonderful reminder that the world is filled with so much beauty.

The next time you go to the beach, spend at least ten minutes trying this exercise. Lie on a blanket or towel. Next, while looking at the water in front of you, soften your gaze or close your eyes if you prefer. Allow yourself to breathe deeply and slowly while taking in your surroundings. How does the wind feel against your skin? What sounds do you hear? Enjoy your beach visit and fully engage your senses. Most likely you'll leave the beach feeling peaceful, refreshed, and more content with life, regardless of how you felt when you arrived.

It's okay if you don't have access to a beach nearby. You can experience the calming effects of ocean waves by listening to an ocean-sounds machine, or you can go online and search for meditative ocean sounds.

Implement a Daily Gratitude Practice

Being grateful for the things in your life not only makes your outlook on life more positive, but also helps give you a sense of peace and calm. Try starting a daily practice of giving thanks for all that is good in your life. There are many ways to implement a daily gratitude practice, and you'll want to choose the one that feels best to you.

You can set a few minutes aside every morning or just before bed every night and simply make a list of the things, people, experiences, and so on in your life that you feel grateful for. You can ask a partner, friend, or family member to do a gratitude practice with you, and you can send each other a text message each day with three things you are feeling grateful for. This is a great way to remain accountable to the practice, and both of you will benefit from all the positive results that feeling grateful provides. If you have family meals around the dinner table, this is a great time for everyone to take turns sharing a couple of things they are grateful for as well.

The moment you start appreciating what you do have instead of dwelling on what you don't have, your entire perspective changes. You start to feel more fulfilled, positive, and happy. Ending your day with a gratitude practice is also a very pleasant and relaxing way to get into a more restful state before bed.

Make a List of Ten Things You Love about Yourself

When was the last time you complimented yourself? When was the last time you said something negative about yourself? Pay attention to your thoughts for a full day and see the way you talk to yourself. Are you being supportive and positive? Or are you criticizing yourself? Criticizing yourself will only bring anxiety, negativity, and stress into your life—all things that are the enemies of calm and rest!

The more you talk negatively to yourself, the more negativity you will manifest in your life. The way you speak to yourself affects your self-image, self-esteem, and so on. In turn, it impacts the results you achieve and how you feel on a regular basis. How can you expect to achieve something positive if you constantly focus on the negative things you see in yourself? Keeping your focus on positivity will help you bring more positive experiences into your life.

Start by listing ten things you love about yourself on a piece of paper. Be honest with yourself, even if this is uncomfortable or feels impossible. The qualities you list don't all have to be physical or about your appearance, just ten things you love about yourself in general! Keep this list handy and read over it every day—actually speak the words aloud and try to embody the feelings as you read them.

Visit a Museum or an Art Gallery

Visiting a museum or an art gallery and looking at different works of art and artifacts can provoke a variety of emotions, including inspiration, joy, and peace. Appreciating the artistic creations of other cultures can lower your stress and anxiety and positively affect your mental health.

At a museum or an art gallery, you can escape the stresses of the day in a quiet, relaxing environment. As with walking in nature or meditating, you simply enjoy living in the present moment and looking at one piece of artwork at a time. It's calming to wander through a museum or gallery unbothered by responsibilities. Visit a museum with exhibits you're excited about and will enjoy. Be mindful when choosing a museum, or at least when choosing which exhibits to explore, that some historical displays may provoke negative emotions and could cause feelings of disgust, anger, or sadness. Do your best to avoid these exhibits so your visit remains uplifting and peaceful.

Take a journal with you so that you can capture your feelings. Sit near an artifact or a piece of art that speaks to you and begin writing in your journal. Write about how it speaks to you and what it makes you feel.

Watch a Funny Movie

Do you want something relaxing to do over the weekend? Plan a movie date with a friend, with your partner, or even by yourself, and choose a funny movie (or two or three) to watch. Laughing helps you relax and distracts you from your worries and stresses. It's no wonder laughter is deemed the best medicine. As you laugh, your body becomes relaxed and less tense. Even if you're angry or frustrated, laughing at a movie will help calm those feelings and make you feel happier.

Choose a funny movie that you've either never seen or have seen and know you love; put on your comfiest pj's; grab your coziest pillow and blanket, a bowl of popcorn, and an ice-cold drink; and settle into "your spot" and hit play! Put your electronics away (yes, even your phone!) and be present in the moment as you watch the movie. You want to really immerse yourself in the movie and allow yourself to feel uplifted, joyful, and relaxed.

Even if you've seen the movie many times, your experience of the movie and the way you feel as a result of watching it in this present and mindful way may surprise you.

Practice Positivity

Most people in our society have a tendency to focus more on negativity than positivity. We have been conditioned to live in constant states of fear, worry, anxiety, scarcity, and lack, and it can feel very unnatural and uncomfortable to suddenly try to think positively throughout the day. Positive thinking requires deliberate daily practice on a consistent basis and then becomes more natural with time.

Living a healthy and happy life full of rest and relaxation will be extremely difficult if you are primarily thinking and feeling negatively. Positive thinking boosts your energy, reduces stress, enhances your sense of well-being, and allows you to relax and rest a lot easier because your mind isn't constantly worrying and ruminating about things that don't feel good.

Try these tips to practice positivity:

* Only watch, listen to, and engage in conversations about things that make you feel good.
* Listen to audiobooks or podcasts on personal development, positive psychology, happiness, and so on.
* Give someone a genuine compliment.
* Practice having an attitude of gratitude.

* Stop taking things personally.
* Focus on the best qualities in others, not the bad qualities.
* Move your body every day. Exercise naturally leads to a more positive mood.
* Surround yourself with positive people.

Play with Your Pet

Pets need playtime to live happy and healthy lives, but did you know that playing with your pet is highly beneficial to your emotional health too? There's a reason why there are emotional support animals! Pets can help you reduce your stress levels by enhancing your serotonin and dopamine levels through playful interaction.

To play with a dog, you can:

* Play fetch with a tennis ball in your backyard.
* Hide treats in a dog puzzle game. Let your dog figure out how to find them.
* Use a rope or plush toy to play tug-of-war.
* Play hide-and-seek with treats.

To play with a cat, you can:

* Wave a feather wand toward your cat and see if the cat can catch it.
* Play with a toy mouse on the floor.
* Get an empty box and put a toy inside. Let your cat climb in and play with it!
* Hide a treat under a plastic cup and see if the cat can find it.

Keep your focus on the present moment as you play with your pet. Take note of how relaxed and joyful you feel when you're being playful, and take the time to play with your pet much more frequently!

Hug a Loved One

One thing you can do to feel more relaxed is to hug a loved one! This doesn't have to be a relationship partner; it can also be a friend or family member! Hugs are among the most comforting and soothing gestures, and they have been scientifically proven to have a positive impact on your health and well-being.

Physical touch is a basic human need, and it is very natural to yearn for touch and affection from others. Human touch increases oxytocin levels, which leads to a feeling of happiness, and lowers cortisol levels (the stress hormone), which promotes feelings of rest and relaxation.

A hug shows someone that you're there for them and helps them feel more safe and secure, comforted, supported, and loved. And the best part is that you experience these same feelings whether you are the one giving or receiving the hug. You want the hug to last for about three seconds to connect with the person more deeply and for both of you to experience the positive benefits.

Some people may not feel comfortable with hugs for various reasons, so be mindful of this when you are about to hug someone for the first time.

Give Yourself a Hug

Yes, self-hugging is a real thing! Hugging yourself sounds silly and may feel a little awkward initially, but hugging yourself has been scientifically proven to be beneficial in many ways, including promoting rest and relaxation.

Physical touch is an innate need of every human being, and we are very naturally drawn to the warmth of affection. However, you don't need another person in order to experience the soothing benefits of being hugged. Your own touch increases oxytocin levels, making you feel happier and less stressed, which allows you to relax and fully rest. Your brain doesn't know the difference between your hugging yourself and your being hugged by someone else, so the hormones are secreted regardless.

You feel more comfortable, supported, and loved when you hug yourself. Anytime you are feeling a little anxious or restless or could really use some soothing touch, just wrap your arms around yourself and squeeze yourself tight or rub your hands up and down the top half of your arms, whatever you find soothing and relaxing. You'll quickly notice that even though it feels somewhat awkward and silly, you really do feel better because of it.

Cuddle Up with a Soft Blanket

Sometimes you just need a good cuddle session to feel more rested and relaxed. If you can't cuddle with a partner, a pet, or someone close to you, you can curl up with a supersoft blanket and cuddle by yourself! If you don't have a favorite cozy blanket to snuggle up with, this is your opportunity to find one you love! Blankets and throws come in an abundance of textures, such as fleece, flannel, faux fur, sherpa, and chenille, so you may want to buy one in person so you can choose the one that feels the most comfortable and cozy to you.

Although cuddling by yourself may not seem as enjoyable or beneficial as cuddling with a loved one, studies have shown that cuddling with a cozy blanket, stuffed animal, or weighted blanket stimulates similar brain activity, which results in feelings of comfort, security, well-being, and love.

Cuddling fosters rest because it causes an increase in oxytocin and a decrease in cortisol, which together promote feelings of relaxation, safety, and security, all of which facilitate sleep. Cuddling also causes an increase in serotonin, "the happy hormone," leading to feelings of happiness and pleasure, which are extremely relaxing.

Find the Silver Lining in Past Challenges

We've all heard the saying "Everything happens for a reason," and although many of us do believe this to be true, during difficult times or painful experiences, we tend to forget this message altogether.

In hindsight, it's much easier to see how being dumped by a significant other, whom we felt we couldn't possibly live without, led to our being single and meeting someone who was a much better match for us; or how getting laid off from a job we really couldn't stand going to opened us up for a much better opportunity and led us down a career path that was much more aligned, fulfilling, and financially rewarding.

Take a moment now to sit and reflect on some painful things you have experienced in your life and the better things that came into your life as a result. This is a very beneficial exercise because it will help you recognize that things are usually working out for our highest good, even when it doesn't feel like it in the moment. Developing this knowing and trust in the universe will help you rest and relax a lot more easily as you face challenges in the future.

Practice Laughter Yoga

Laughter yoga is a style of yoga that promotes deliberate laughter through a series of movement and breathing exercises. Laughter yoga is typically practiced in a group setting and has become increasingly popular online. The intention of laughter yoga is to help you remove any internal judgment you feel toward yourself and to let go, relax, and take yourself less seriously.

A trained laughing yoga instructor leads the group through various exercises that promote laughter, playfulness, and joy. The teacher will deliberately begin to laugh, and because laughter is contagious, class participants will naturally start laughing as well. It won't take long until everyone in the class is giggling uncontrollably. There is nothing quite like it, and it brings out the inner child within you.

For most adults, their responsibilities tend to take precedence over just having fun and laughing. The purpose of laughter yoga is to encourage laughter and positivity. Laughter yoga also includes controlled breathing, which helps you better manage stress. Controlled breathing allows your body to absorb more oxygen, which activates the parasympathetic nervous system, your body's innate relaxation system.

It's hard to feel anything other than joyful, relaxed, and carefree in a laughter yoga class!

Visualize Your Ideal Self and Ideal Life

Visualizing your ideal life and ideal self can be a very enjoyable and relaxing experience and can help you design your life with clarity and purpose. People rarely take the time to consider how they would rather be living. If you pause to think through how your ideal life and ideal self would look and feel, you can begin taking inspired action to become your ideal self and create your ideal life over time. This isn't about unrealistic fantasizing; the purpose is to imagine an ideal life that is attainable.

Start by answering the following questions in a notebook: Where and how would you be living? What would you spend your time doing? How would you feel most often? Who would you spend your time with?

After writing out the answers, sit in a comfortable position and close your eyes. Visualize waking up one morning in your ideal life, as your ideal self. In vivid detail imagine living out the entire day, moment by moment, through your ideal self's eyes, and try to fully embody the feelings as though you are experiencing this ideal reality in real time. Practice this visualization daily to relax and reprogram your mind.

Acknowledge Your Current Emotions

The ability to notice how you're feeling at any given time will improve your emotional well-being. As you begin to experience greater self-awareness, you will become better at noticing how you are feeling at any given moment. The sooner you can recognize that you are experiencing negative feelings, the easier it is to figure out what contributed to them.

Although emotions can feel overwhelming, they provide you with valuable information, so they should not be ignored. The root cause of emotions is often something much larger than the present situation. Identifying why you feel a certain way will allow you to understand your feelings better.

Begin by sitting or lying down, closing your eyes, and taking a few deep breaths. Ask yourself what you are currently feeling and allow yourself to feel it fully. Notice how your body is responding. Is your heart beating faster? Do you feel tension anywhere? Consider asking yourself when you first noticed feeling this way and see if you can determine the reason behind your emotions. Don't judge your feelings, just witness and allow them.

The more present you are willing and able to be in any given moment, the more relaxed you will feel.

Stop and Smell the Flowers

We all need occasional reminders to slow down and become aware of and appreciative of all the incredible things in our life. So why not literally stop and smell the flowers every day?

Make this a spiritual practice you can do every day! It's an opportunity to appreciate and savor the beauty nature has to offer. The next time you see flowers, take it as a sign to stop and smell them. Think of one thing you're grateful for at that very moment as you stop to smell the flowers, even if you just feel grateful that you noticed the flowers!

Amid the hustle and bustle of our busy lives, it's easy to miss opportunities such as these. But as we begin cultivating more self-awareness and become more present and mindful as we move through our lives, it can feel very relaxing and rewarding to take note of the beautiful things all around us and feel appreciation for our awareness of them.

Taking brief moments here and there to slow down and be present and to feel happy and grateful for the little things in life is a wonderful way to add little moments of rest and relaxation into your day!

Let Go of Toxic Relationships

Take a moment to reflect on your relationships. Are any of them emotionally draining, hard to deal with, or just unhealthy? Are you experiencing constant negativity and feeling unsupported? If so, you might be in a toxic relationship. Negativity in any relationship doesn't serve anyone well, and toxicity could reduce your self-confidence and increase stress.

Think about whether you want to communicate how you feel before you walk away entirely from a negative relationship. You can express your unwillingness to tolerate toxic behavior by establishing boundaries with that person. Detail what you are not willing to accept. Perhaps there was a misunderstanding. Nevertheless, you should follow your intuition if you feel stepping away is best for your emotional health. The presence of negativity in your life every day does not serve you.

To maintain good emotional health, you must have fulfilling and joyful relationships. Cherish those relationships and keep them close to your heart. Make sure you take care of your emotional well-being and surround yourself with people who will support you, love you, and improve your life. Protect your energy and your emotional health! You will rest easier and feel much more relaxed after cutting toxic ties.

Tell Yourself "I Love You"

As you begin to gain more self-awareness, you may be surprised to realize just how often you are beating yourself up in your mind. Becoming aware of the negativity you are constantly spewing is the first step in changing those habitual patterns, and that's all they are! Getting into the habit of speaking kindlier to yourself will benefit you and your inner peace tremendously.

You may think that saying "I love you" to yourself is silly, or too simplistic, and won't make any difference. These thoughts are very common. We tend to have a lot of resistance to doing this. It's okay! Allow the thoughts and feelings to arise and do it anyway!

Commit to looking in a mirror and telling yourself "I love you" every single day. Take a few minutes to just be there with yourself. Don't rush through it, don't just think it, but speak the words aloud and really look deeply into your eyes. When most of us look at ourselves in the mirror, we are extremely critical, noticing all kinds of perceived flaws. If you focus on looking deeply into your eyes, everything else will fade away.

Over time, these words will become very soothing and relaxing. Give it a try!

Let Yourself Cry

Are you aware that letting yourself cry can help you cope with pain? Tears soothe your emotional state by releasing oxytocin. So, allow yourself to cry if you feel the need to. It's important to fully feel all your emotions and to freely express them.

Understand that this is a natural part of being human. If you are experiencing a significant life event, more stress than usual, and a mixture of emotions, crying can benefit you. Those trapped emotions can be released through tears. If you let yourself cry, you'll feel more relaxed because you won't be trying so hard to keep it all bottled in. You can allow your body and mind to relax while experiencing all the emotions.

Watching a movie that makes you emotional can be an excellent way to release some of your pent-up emotions. Have you ever watched something and been surprised by how strongly you were affected by it? Did it make you sob or cry uncontrollably? Some sort of emotional block may have been released and the feelings couldn't help but pour out. You can also experience tears of joy through watching a movie. Either way, it can be very therapeutic and relaxing.

Have That Hard Conversation

Is there a tough conversation that you've been putting off because it feels awkward or uncomfortable to talk about? Do you just keep avoiding the conversation, or maybe even the person altogether? Stuffing down your feelings is a sure way to increase your stress and anxiety and keep you from feeling restful and relaxed. It's so important to be open and honest about what you are feeling and then be able to express it.

Feeling strongly about something and forcing yourself to keep it bottled in "to keep the peace" is extremely exhausting, both physically and mentally. This is especially true if you live together and must see each other every day. Putting the well-being of the other person, or the well-being of the relationship in general, ahead of your own well-being can be very detrimental.

Although the conversation may be uncomfortable, finally expressing your feelings openly and honestly will help you relax and rest so much easier. Remember, having a difficult conversation does not mean that the relationship is doomed. Conflict is natural in any relationship. Healthy relationships still experience occasional conflict. What makes the relationship healthy is both partners' ability to freely express themselves openly and honestly. Communication is a vital component to any healthy relationship.

Do a Noting Meditation

Meditation techniques are often described as being either calming or insightful. The intention of a calming meditation is simply to cultivate a quieter, more peaceful state of mind, and to strengthen concentration. Most calming meditation practices involve focusing on something specific such as your breath, a mantra, or a physical object and then returning your focus to that subject whenever you notice your mind has wandered off. Alternatively, people who practice insight meditation often set an intention to transform their minds by developing qualities such as personal insight, wisdom, and compassion.

A noting meditation is a type of insight meditation. You can practice a noting meditation in two ways: by focusing on your breath or simply sitting quietly in stillness. All this technique involves is conscious awareness, specifically "noting" what's distracting the mind. As soon as you notice that you've been distracted by a thought or an emotion and that you've lost your awareness of the breath or the stillness, "note" the thought or feeling to restore awareness, to create a bit of space, and to learn more about your habitual thought patterns, tendencies, and conditioning.

Sitting quietly in stillness is one of the most restful and relaxing things you can do.

Scream and Release

Have you ever allowed yourself to scream at the top of your lungs? If so, you know how satisfying it feels! When you shout, your body releases the "feel good" chemicals you crave. Screaming can be very cathartic and healing! Science has even proven that screaming is good for your well-being. Unfortunately, societal norms don't allow for random outbursts of screaming your lungs out.

Throughout our lives, we've been taught that we shouldn't express our anger or negative emotions, and because of this many of us have a lifetime's worth of negative energy stored in our bodies. Screaming helps to release those suppressed emotions and can help you rest and relax so much more because you are no longer bogged down with all that negative energy.

However, understandably, human screams immediately activate fear responses deep in the minds of other humans when they hear them. You need to be mindful of this whenever you decide to implement a screaming release practice and take necessary precautions to ensure that no one else will hear you. The most ideal time to let yourself scream is when you're alone in your car and can find a safe, secluded place to scream it out!

Connect with Online Groups

If your idea of resting and relaxing is to lie on the couch and mindlessly scroll through social media (not recommended, but we get it!), it would serve you well to at least be conscious of the type of accounts you follow and the groups you are a part of. Like anything else, the Internet is full of both positive and negative influences, and your experience of it is entirely up to you.

Consciously choose to follow only positive, inspiring, and uplifting accounts so the content you are scrolling through is beneficial, and not detrimental to your mental health and well-being like the content posted on the news channels' accounts. Instead of just scrolling through whatever content the particular social media platform has determined is important and relevant, be mindful in what you choose to see. If you notice negative emotions arising from a particular profile, unfollow that person or group!

Joining *Facebook* groups or similar types of groups on other platforms based on your interests, passions, and life pursuits can be a wonderful way to connect with other like-minded people and make friends all over the world!

Lying around scrolling through content that evokes only good feelings can be quite relaxing!

Write a Poem

Writing a poem is a relaxing and creative way to facilitate honest expression. Poetry allows you to freely express yourself by using lively phrases, rhythmic language, and colorful descriptions. As a therapeutic form of writing, poetry provides a creative outlet for allowing feelings to surface. Releasing emotions through artistic expression is very soothing.

You can explore different types of poetry if you think you might want to try a more structured type such as a haiku, sonnet, or limerick. You may recall learning about these kinds of poetry in school but don't really remember any of the specifics. It could be fun to refresh your memory on some of them and see what you feel inspired to create.

However, if structure isn't really your thing and you'd rather write free verse poetry, do that! This is also a fun and liberating way to let your creativity flow. When you are writing, don't monitor yourself and don't hold back. Remember, this is all about being raw and honest rather than perfect!

Find a quiet, comfortable place, sit down with a notebook and pen, and let your imagination run wild! Soft instrumental background music may make the experience even more relaxing and enjoyable.

Release Judgment

Releasing judgment is so beneficial to your mental health and well-being! Constantly feeling critical of yourself and others is not a very peaceful way to live. Anytime you are feeling judgmental, you are not relaxed. Judgment is a signal that you have unresolved negative feelings within you.

Making judgments about yourself and others will not serve you; they will only prevent you from living a positive life. Whether or not you mean to be judgmental, you're only expressing how you feel about yourself when you judge someone else. Whenever you catch yourself feeling critical or judgmental, stop and ask yourself if you are feeling triggered in some way.

For example, if you notice yourself judging someone for purchasing a brand-new car, pause and ask yourself what these uncomfortable feelings are really reflecting to you. Are you not able to afford a brand-new car because you don't manage your money well? Does the idea of money in general stir up uncomfortable feelings for you? Starting to become more aware of your thoughts and feelings and doing the inner work necessary to uncover and overcome some deep-seated emotional blocks is a wonderful way to experience more rest and relaxation.

Learn to Let Go

If you want to experience more rest and relaxation, you must learn to let go! Truthfully, there are very few things in life you have control over. Finally coming to this realization after a lifelong quest to be in control of everything (and everyone!) might just feel like a relief.

The easiest and quickest way to begin letting go is to stop and ask yourself if whatever is troubling you in that moment is something you can change. If the answer is yes, change it. If the answer is no, let it go!

For example, say you work for a small, privately owned company and your boss doesn't give you the day off work on the Friday before a Saturday holiday, or the Monday after a Sunday holiday, like many corporate jobs do. This makes you mad and you think it's unfair.

Ask yourself, can I change this? You can choose to work somewhere else, but if you continue working for this company and this boss, it's out of your control. Letting go and not allowing it to cause you to feel mad or resentful is a much more peaceful way to live.

Be Yourself

One of the most freeing feelings we can experience as humans is just simply being ourselves.

If you have the courage to be true to yourself and live authentically, you will find inner peace. Doing whatever makes you happy and expressing your authentic self unapologetically is a very relaxing and enjoyable way to live.

Wearing the clothes that make you feel good, eating the foods that make you happy, and speaking truthfully about your opinions and beliefs, regardless of what anyone else thinks, is so liberating.

You must know that you are worthy and deserving of being accepted and loved exactly as you are. When you focus your energy and attention on the things you love that light you up, you will no longer compare yourself to others because you will be too happy to care what anyone else is doing.

Take pride in your unique characteristics. Ignoring those special qualities and trying to blend in is the worst thing you can do. It's exhausting trying to live your life as anyone other than your true self. Your life will feel completely out of alignment. The more you fall in love with your authentic self, the more others will too!

Prioritize Self-Compassion

Do you put a lot of pressure on yourself? Do you always strive for perfection? Are you overly critical of yourself? If so, you may want to start feeling some self-compassion! Self-compassion is about giving yourself the same level of understanding, kindness, and love you would give to a good friend.

The most important thing about practicing self-compassion is that you honor and accept your humanness. Self-compassion has many benefits, including:

* Provides support during times of stress
* Enhances accountability
* Encourages living a more active and healthier lifestyle
* Stabilizes emotional well-being
* Ensures others are cared for
* Boosts resilience after major life crises

To practice more self-compassion, start with the following:

* Take good care of your emotional health by keeping a self-compassion journal.
* Show gratitude for the blessings in your life. Ask yourself what you're grateful for every day.

* Avoid judging yourself for past mistakes and be kind to yourself. Rather than dwelling on the past, commit to learning and growing.
* Practice saying positive affirmations to yourself in the mirror every morning.

If you start replacing your old negative habits of self-judgment and self-criticism with self-compassion and self-love, you will quickly recognize noticeable improvements in how peaceful and relaxed you feel.

Learn to Forgive

Your physical and mental health will improve tremendously if you learn to forgive. You will also feel so much lighter and more relaxed when you're no longer dragging around old pain and suffering. When you hold on to painful and traumatic experiences from your past, you tend to think the people who harmed you are somehow paying for the pain and suffering they caused you. Unfortunately, they aren't the ones holding on to the negative feelings of hurt, pain, suffering, betrayal, anger, and resentment; you are. So, you are the one experiencing the innumerable negative consequences as a result, not them.

The most important thing to realize is that forgiveness is never about the other person. It's not about letting someone "off the hook" or condoning that person's behavior. Forgiveness is always only about you and your healing. The other person never even needs to know that you have extended forgiveness. It's not done for that person's peace of mind, but only for your own! Forgiveness is about freeing yourself from unnecessary suffering. This requires acceptance. You must accept that what happened, happened. You cannot go back and change it, but you can decide to rise above it and no longer allow it to affect your life.

Start a Family Worry Jar

Writing down and disposing of negative thoughts can be very helpful. Using a worry jar is an excellent way to manage your stress. It's all about gaining awareness of your thoughts and feelings, writing them down, and releasing them (or at least getting them out of your mind and into the jar).

The simple act of writing things down is often enough to stop them from endlessly swirling around in your mind all day, which can be mentally exhausting! This practice not only gets them out of your mind but locks them away in a jar where they can affect you only if you allow them to!

All you need are a large jar with a lid, some scrap paper, and a pen. Then anytime you notice an unhelpful, unhealthy, or even unpleasant thought creep into your mind, go to the worry jar and write down the thoughts and feelings on a piece of paper. Crumble the paper into a ball, place it in the jar, and close the lid tightly. As you do this, set the intention of releasing the thoughts from your mind.

Notice how much more relaxed and peaceful you feel without so much negativity filling your head.

Practice Box Breathing

There are many different forms of deep breathing exercises. One form of deep breathing that has been found to be particularly helpful with relaxation is box breathing. Box breathing is often used for stress management and can be practiced before, during, and/or after the stressful experience.

The practice consists of four simple steps, each done to a count of four. For this practice, you want to be seated in a chair with your feet flat on the floor. Rest your hands in your lap with your palms facing up, and make sure you are sitting up nice and straight, which allows you to take nice deep breaths.

1. Inhale slowly and deeply through your nose to the slow count of four (in your head). Focus on the feeling of the air filling your lungs.
2. Hold your breath for another slow count of four.
3. Exhale slowly and deeply through your mouth to the slow count of four. Focus on the feeling of the air leaving your lungs.
4. Hold your breath for another slow count of four (simply avoid inhaling or exhaling).
5. Repeat this cycle a total of four times.

You can utilize this practice anytime you want to rest or relax.

Paint Inspirational Stones

Inspirational stones are stones with inspirational words or phrases painted on them. Creating them can be a fun and relaxing project to do alone, with children, or with friends!

Oftentimes, inspirational stones are placed in gardens, around sidewalks, or along walking trails or running paths, and these tend to be larger in size. If you've ever come across one during a neighborhood stroll, it likely brightened your day. These colorful stones can easily uplift your spirits.

You can also paint much smaller stones—stones that fit comfortably in your palm—and set them on a dresser, an entryway table, or a bathroom counter for a little sprinkle of inspiration throughout your home.

For this project you will need an assortment of smooth stones, acrylic paint, paintbrushes, and a waterproof paint sealer (if you are placing them outdoors). Clean and dry the stones if necessary and then let the paint and inspiration flow!

You can write single words such as "peace," "love," or "believe," or positive affirmations such as "choose joy" or "I am enough." Decorate the stones in any way that makes you feel good, and you will spread that same positive energy with others when they see your works of art.

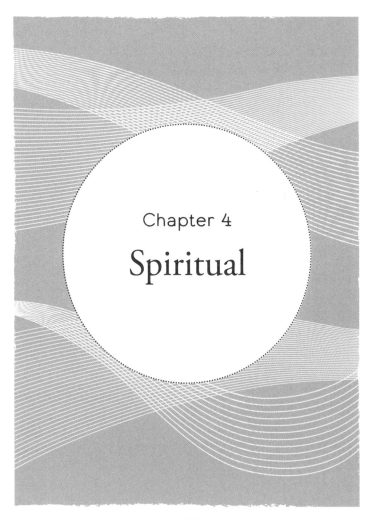

Chapter 4

Spiritual

This chapter will help you learn ways to get in touch with your spiritual side while prioritizing rest and relaxation. The activities in this chapter aren't about a specific religion or practice; they're about tapping in to your own higher power and innate connection with the universe. Spirituality gives you a sense of connection with something bigger than yourself.

The activities in this chapter will help you rediscover your true self. With activities ranging from practicing grounding and watching the sunrise to spending time alone and volunteering for an important cause, they will connect you with nature, your community, and your soul's purpose.

As you practice spirituality, you begin to realize that there are only so many things within your control, and taking time to rest and be in the present moment can be one of the most beneficial ways to experience life. Everyone experiences spirituality differently, but engaging in relaxing spiritual activities will help you reconnect with your soul and trust your inner guidance. As a result, you'll feel more in touch with the world around you and find a greater sense of peace in your daily life.

Practice Grounding

Grounding is a therapeutic technique used to realign your energy with the earth. Something quite magical happens when you simply touch your bare feet to the earth. A transfer of energy occurs. You have a positive charge, and the earth has a negative charge, and when you connect your bare feet directly with the ground, the earth helps you release excess energy. This makes grounding feel very relaxing and rejuvenating.

To practice grounding, you just need to find a safe, clear space in your yard, at a local park, or on a nearby beach. Any open area with grass, dirt, or sand can be a great option for grounding. With bare feet, stand tall with your spine in proper alignment and your feet shoulder width apart. Relax your gaze or, if you feel comfortable, close your eyes. Bring your attention to your feet and really focus on the feeling of the soles of your feet connecting with the ground as you breathe slowly and deeply. You might feel the energy from the ground moving upward through your feet and to the rest of your body. Taking a few minutes to feel grounded every day is a wonderful way to rest and relax.

Lie on the Beach

There's just something about the peaceful waves, salty breeze, and soft sand that makes the beach so soothing. Naturally, this makes the beach a wonderful place to rest and relax.

If the sand isn't too hot, you can lie directly on it if you want a deeper connection with the earth. Of course, you can always lay down a blanket or towel if you prefer. Be sure to always protect yourself from the sun with proper clothing and sunscreen. You can also use an umbrella or a beach tent if you don't want to be directly in the sun.

Once you've set up your beach space, let yourself enjoy your surroundings. Lie down on your back, either directly on the sand or on your towel, and turn your focus to the sound of the crashing waves. Take slow, deep breaths to relax even more. As long as you're protected from the sun, you can allow yourself to drift off to sleep.

After your beach nap, you'll feel rejuvenated and refreshed. You'll feel better spiritually as you'll be more in touch with yourself and the nature around you. The beach is always there for you anytime you want to relax or rest.

Sit Outside and Listen to Nature Sounds

That feeling of calm you experience when you hear birds chirping or rain pounding on the rooftop isn't all in your head. Listening to nature sounds decreases the body's sympathetic response, which causes that "fight-or-flight" feeling and increases the parasympathetic response, or "rest-and-digest" response, which helps the body relax. This leads to a reduction in anxiety, depression, and stress. It also lowers blood pressure, improves concentration, and instills a general feeling of calmness and well-being.

To reap the soothing benefits of nature sounds, follow these steps:

1. Go outside and find a nice spot to sit, perhaps against a tree.
2. Close your eyes and take a few deep breaths while you tune in to your surroundings.
3. Turn your attention to all the delightful sounds you can hear, from the leaves rustling in the wind to birds singing in the trees.

4. Simply notice the sounds, allowing your attention to wander from one sound to another. Practice this for five to ten minutes.
5. When you're ready, open your eyes and notice how good your body and mind feel.

You can also experience the benefits of nature sounds by using a nature sound machine, using a nature sound app, or listening to nature sounds online.

Do a Gratitude Meditation

Gratitude meditation is simply the practice of reflecting on the things in your life you're grateful for. It's about fully experiencing the feeling of appreciation, rather than the intellectual idea. Appreciation is a heartwarming feeling that encourages you to be more present, and a deep sense of gratitude helps you connect to something larger than yourself, whether that be to other people, nature, or the universe at large. The more familiar these feelings become, the more frequently you're likely to experience them.

Gratitude meditation is like relaxation meditation (see Chapter 2); however, instead of focusing on your breath, you will be focusing on the things, people, and experiences in your life that you feel grateful for. You can do this anytime and anywhere! You can incorporate it into your morning or bedtime routine or even do it while you are standing in line at the grocery store. All it requires is slowing down, becoming present, and focusing on how grateful you feel for a loved one, a steady paycheck, your healthy body, anything!

Taking a few minutes each day to consciously focus on appreciation feels so peaceful and relaxing, and the long-term benefits of this consistent practice foster greater health and happiness.

Watch the Sunset

In today's hustle culture, everyone is always so busy rushing from one thing to the next, distracted by their devices, going through their daily routine on autopilot, completely unaware of much of the beauty the world has to offer.

Most people live in places where the sun rises and sets every day, yet very few ever take the time to slow down and become present enough to consciously watch the sunset. There's just something about a sunset that feels so serene and relaxing. Not to mention that admiring the rich colors of the expansive sky spanning as far as the eye can see, in all directions, gives you a sense of the vastness of the universe, and at the same time makes you feel a deeper connection with it.

Mindfully watching the sunset is one of the most awe-inspiring and spiritually fulfilling experiences we can have as human beings. Nevertheless, this experience is freely available to most of us, almost every day, and we never even notice it.

This evening, go outside just before sunset and take ten minutes to slow down, relax, and mindfully watch the sunset (without distractions) and just enjoy its magnificence.

Watch the Sunrise

Do you typically wake up before the sun? Whether it's because you must wake up early for work or you just naturally wake up early, taking some me time for yourself in the mornings (before anyone else in your household is awake) is a wonderfully relaxing way to begin the day.

One way to make this me time even more relaxing and enjoyable is by watching the sunrise. Are you able to view the sunrise from your yard? Even if you cannot see the sunrise over the horizon from your home, just witnessing the sky transition from color to color and watching the sky becoming brighter and brighter as the sun rises can be very relaxing and uplifting.

Wrap up in a cozy blanket, take your favorite morning drink outside with you, and wake up with the sun. There's something so peaceful about watching the sunrise and acknowledging a fresh start and a new beginning. This is a perfect way to mindfully prepare for the day ahead.

Wake up with the sun tomorrow morning! Even if that means waking up earlier than usual just to catch the sunrise, you might find that it's even more enjoyable than sleeping would've been!

Lie in Savasana

One of the most beloved parts of a yoga class is Savasana. Savasana is a yoga pose in which you lie down flat on your back on your yoga mat. This pose is traditionally done at the end of a yoga class and typically lasts anywhere from thirty seconds to fifteen minutes.

With this pose, yoga students can experience deep relaxation and a profound spiritual experience. It is recommended that students close their eyes, relax their arms by their sides, and let their feet rest at the bottom corners of the yoga mat. Yoga teachers sometimes wrap their students in blankets for extra comfort, or play soothing music during this time of class and guide students through a full-body scan or meditation. This pose is so relaxing that many students even drift off to sleep.

Whenever you're feeling the need to relax your body and mind or want to get in touch with your emotions and spirit, lie down flat on the ground on a blanket or yoga mat and turn on your favorite yoga music or a meditation playlist, or just lie there in silence. If you have obligations and worry about falling asleep, set a timer for yourself.

Write a Love Letter to Yourself

Writing letters to yourself can be a beautiful way to express self-love. Although it may feel silly or awkward initially and you may even notice some resistance, the process of writing kind words to yourself will create a deeper connection with your inner being, which will make you feel more at peace and calm.

There are many ways you can write a love letter to yourself. There are no rules or restrictions; you just want to make sure that you are focusing on positive feelings toward yourself throughout the writing process. Focus on feeling self-acceptance, self-compassion, and self-love primarily. You can write it however you want but here are two possible ideas:

* You can write a letter to your inner child and tell them all the things they (you) needed to hear when they (you) were younger, but never heard.
* You can write it as your future self; for example, the seventy-five-year-old version of you can write it to your present-day self and fill you in on all the amazing and beautiful experiences your life was filled with between now and age seventy-five.

Find a quiet space where you won't be disturbed, a notebook, and your favorite pen, and start writing! Fill yourself with love and enjoy this therapeutic and relaxing experience.

Try Watercolor Painting

Watercolor paintings are beautiful to look at and peaceful to create. Painting can be a profoundly spiritual and therapeutic experience! Painting with watercolors and watching the colors flow and interact with one another can be very soothing. Fully immersing yourself in the creative process allows you to be present in the moment and let go of everything else for a little while. This is a wonderful way to relax and allow your mind to rest.

You can create an abstract painting, a beautiful landscape, whatever you want! You'll need watercolor paper, watercolor paints, a palette, paintbrushes, water, cups, paper towels, and a flat surface or an easel.

As you paint, tune in to your inner world. Allow the thoughts and feelings to come and go with no judgment, just awareness. As you're painting, feel love and gratitude for your inspired creation. The purpose of painting is to enjoy the creative process, not just the finished piece. It's about authentic expression and the expansion experienced through the creative process. The beautiful part about painting is that there are no rules, just an opportunity to freely express yourself. It's simply a matter of being present and creating whatever comes through you.

Do a Sound Bath Meditation

Different cultures have been healing bodies through sound for thousands of years. A sound bath is a meditative experience in which those in attendance are "bathed" in sound waves. The sound waves are produced by various sources, including healing instruments such as gongs, singing bowls, percussion, chimes, rattles, tuning forks, and even the human voice itself.

The sounds don't create a catchy melody or rhythm or anything like that—the sounds aren't supposed to sound repetitive in any way because you don't want the brain to recognize and latch on to a repeated beat. You want the participant's brain to let go. The intention of a sound bath is really to change and help balance the participant's energy.

You can look for sound bath meditations at your local yoga and meditation studios, or you can find them online. There are even sound bath apps you can use to experience this healing technique.

Sound baths have been proven to provide physical and mental health benefits as well as improvements in overall well-being. Sound baths are a wonderful way to rest and relax so give them a try!

Practice Chanting "Om"

If you've taken a yoga class, you might have heard "om" chanted three times to end class. From yoga's beginnings, this mantra has been a vital element.

"Om" has three sounds and is pronounced "aaa-uuu-mmm." It creates a deep vibration in your body, bringing you into conscious awareness. Because of the vibration it creates, chanting "om" relaxes your body and mind and attracts positive energy to your life. This chant improves concentration and focus. It can help you achieve deep relaxation by putting you into a meditative state. The soul is allowed to rest, and you can become in tune with your energy.

Chanting this mantra can help you sleep better too! If you chant "om" as part of your bedtime meditation, you will notice how it helps clear your mind and prepares you for sleep.

To prepare for your chanting session, find a quiet place. Sit comfortably with a tall, straight upper body. Close your eyes and inhale deeply and then slowly exhale. After your next inhale, begin saying "om" slowly as you're exhaling. Chant the mantra three times, and then sit with your eyes closed as you feel the vibration through your body.

Play a Singing Bowl

Have you tried meditating with a singing bowl? Singing bowls make soothing vibrational sounds that you can feel within your entire body and soul. They're a great addition to your meditation practice or whenever you want to ease your mind from all the thoughts and to-do lists. The sound of singing bowls is deeply relaxing for the spirit and can help clear negative energy. It will allow you to sleep more soundly and promote more rest in your life.

You can find handmade singing bowls for sale in specialty online stores or meditation studios. Trying the various options in person allows you to determine which one resonates with you the most. Various sizes are available, and each size has its own tone and effect.

To make the bowl "sing," you need to use the wooden mallet that comes with it while holding the bowl in your other hand. The wooden mallet should be glided gently along the bowl's outer edges. A beautiful vibration will begin to occur.

While listening to the peaceful sounds, pay close attention to your breath and focus on the present moment. Allow your eyes to close to feel the sound vibrations eliminate anxiety and stress from your body.

Light a Scented Candle

Create a peaceful environment in your home by lighting a scented candle! The flickering light of a candle in a dimly lit room gives off the most relaxing ambience. Candles, in general, create a peaceful atmosphere that encourages rest and meditation and can be beneficial as part of your spiritual practice. Candles scented with essential oils can make relaxing even more effective because these aromatherapy candles can profoundly affect mood, stress reduction, productivity, and overall well-being.

When you burn a candle with essential oils, your energy will become calmer and more positive. Candles with lavender essential oil have relaxing and stress-relieving properties that help you rest and sleep better. If you're looking for other calming scents, look for candles with chamomile, jasmine, or rose essential oils.

Light a scented candle to help create a relaxing atmosphere in your home before meditating, journaling, tarot reading, practicing yoga, taking a bubble bath, and so on.

If you are sensitive to scents, unscented candles can also be relaxing. If you are planning on an activity or meditation where you may drift off to sleep, battery-operated candles are a safe and recommended option. Many battery-operated candles even have very realistic flickering flames!

Plant Flowers in Your Garden

Do you want an easy way to create a more relaxing environment? Then plant some beautiful flowers in your garden! When flowers surround you, your spirit is connected to the earth's beauty.

You can spend more time in your garden if you plan it around the space you use most. If you spend more of your time indoors, create a small area with potted plants inside. Consider adding flowers to your outdoor living area if you spend most of your time outdoors.

The rose is one of the flowers that promote relaxation. A rose garden will allow you to stop and smell the roses at any time! Sunflowers, azaleas, and peonies are instant mood boosters, making them an excellent fit for a space where you spend a lot of time. Planting jasmine flowers will make you feel grounded and calm.

Flowers with colors that promote a positive mood and relaxation can be beneficial to include in your space. Consider blue tones to create a restful space and yellow colors for more energy. The options are endless, and every flower has its own distinct benefits and beauty.

Spend Time Alone

Have you ever wished you had more time for yourself? In a time when we are all digitally connected through social media and our phones, it can feel like we never have time just for ourselves. So, stepping away from all the noise and creating a quiet oasis is imperative to fully rest and relax.

Taking some time to be alone is healthy and can be deeply fulfilling. Solitude is beneficial for your spiritual well-being, mental health, and creativity. It's your chance to focus on what makes your soul happy instead of focusing on all the other responsibilities you have in your life. If you constantly focus on the world around you, you may lose the potential to evolve and grow spiritually.

Being alone does not have to be boring! Here are some enjoyable activities you can do by yourself:

* Listen to a guided meditation
* Bake cookies
* Go for a long walk in your neighborhood
* Gaze at the stars at night
* Take a long bath
* Read a new book
* Dance to your favorite song
* Take a course you've wanted to take

Find Your True Purpose

As humans, one of the most challenging and confusing things is figuring out the meaning of our lives and what we want to do in life. We are often told that we are supposed to find our true purpose in life and do something meaningful. This kind of thinking can put a lot of pressure on simply living and prevent us from living a peaceful life.

While it is important to find what you enjoy doing, it is essential to realize that you are meant to appreciate the act of existence, and there is nothing more that you need to do in life other than to simply be yourself.

Indigenous teachings remind us that humans are a part of the same cycle of being as plants and animals, who give and receive with each other to thrive. There is fulfillment in simply existing within this life cycle. The realization that your purpose is to simply exist, like plants and animals, is truly enlightening. It feels freeing and takes away the stress of figuring out what you are "meant to do" during your lifetime. When you come to terms with this thought, your soul will find peace knowing that you are always in your purpose.

Volunteer for a Cause That's Important to You

Volunteering for a cause that's near and dear to your heart can be one of the most fulfilling experiences and can provide a greater sense of purpose. Knowing you have helped someone is a very rewarding feeling. The positive feelings volunteering will evoke within you will minimize your stress, help you rest more easily, and make you feel better overall.

You become more empathetic when you volunteer. It's easier to relate to others' struggles when you witness them firsthand. Working as a volunteer improves morale, fosters gratitude, and provides a sense of spiritual fulfillment.

Make a list of the top five organizations that mean the most to you. Ask yourself if you want to work with children, animals, adults, or an environmental project. Check each organization's website for local events. Another great option is to do a direct search for nearby volunteer opportunities. You will likely find several organizations to choose from. A few options are animal shelters, soup kitchens, and women's shelters.

Set a goal for yourself to volunteer more. Determine how often you'd like to volunteer and start scheduling events accordingly. You can invite friends and family to join you. Have fun and give with your heart!

Read a Personal Development Book

Enhance your life experience by reading personal development books! Books in this genre can help you connect more deeply with yourself and can help you start to develop a deeper understanding about humanity in general. Reading is a great stress reliever, and reading personal development books will help you see yourself and the world around you in a more positive light.

Personal development books are very introspective. They often include writing exercises and journaling prompts that encourage self-reflection and ask you to apply what you are learning in the book to your own life experiences. Reading these inspirational books is a great way to get in touch with your soul and learn how to live more positively!

You can explore so many topics in this genre, such as relationships, productivity, spirituality, time management, health, and mindfulness. Select a book you are eager to read and a topic you would like to learn more about.

Keep a self-development book on your nightstand if you want to increase your spiritual connection and relaxation. You can feel better when you begin and end your day with a few minutes of reading. Sit back, relax, and read an inspiring book!

Step Outside of Your Comfort Zone

If you stay in your comfort zone for too long, you won't likely experience spiritual or mental growth. Trying new things helps you grow and learn as well as connect with your soul. When you try something new and realize there is no reason to be fearful, you will also introduce more relaxation into your life.

To do this, you first need to ask yourself what you consider to be out of your comfort zone. Then, try the following:

* Repeat a mantra every day that challenges your current thoughts. "I am confident." "I am fearless."
* Make small changes to your daily routine, like going to bed earlier and waking up earlier.
* Try something new every week. Try a new movie or book genre, or a different spa treatment.
* Start a unique hobby.
* Visit a new town.
* Take a course on something you've always wanted to learn but haven't.

So, are you ready to try something new? Introducing new ways to rest requires you to step out of your comfort zone. The more you do it, the easier it will get. Don't run away from discomfort; embrace it instead! This will significantly enhance your happiness and ability to rest.

Spend Time in Prayer

Do you pray regularly? Do you pray only during difficult and troubling times? Have you never prayed before? Implementing a daily practice of prayer may help you feel better mentally and connect more deeply with your spirit. No matter your religion, spending time in prayer will strengthen your spirituality and help you feel more peaceful and relaxed.

Spending more time in prayer will also enhance the connection you feel with yourself, your god, and the universe in general.

Commit to implementing this daily practice now and choose a specific time of day for prayer. Creating new habits is a lot easier when you combine them with something you already do consistently, such as journaling, drinking coffee, or brushing your teeth. So, for example, if you commit to praying every day while you are enjoying your morning coffee, this will help you develop the new habit of praying.

Also, the amount of time you spend praying does not matter, but the intention of your prayer does. Trust your intuition and spend only as much time in prayer as feels right to you.

Over time, you will likely notice gradual positive changes occurring in your life because of this practice.

Meditate on a Personal Mantra

Mantras are repetitive sounds used to penetrate the depths of the unconscious mind through vibration. Mantras are vibrated through chanting aloud, through mental practice, or by listening to them. Mantras are an important part of the yogic and meditation practices. When you meditate, you can silently use mantras as your point of focus.

Think about a mantra you'd like to tell yourself more often. What do you currently need more of in your life? If you need more rest, some mantras you can meditate on are "I am at peace," "I am calm," or "I trust that I have everything I need within me." Choose a mantra you feel spiritually connected to and use it as your point of focus in meditation.

This will be much like the relaxation meditation from Chapter 2. However, instead of focusing on and counting your breaths, you are going to be focusing on saying the mantra, either silently in your mind or aloud if you prefer, repeatedly, until the timer goes off.

If you meditate on the mantra "I am calm" and you truly feel it as you repeatedly say it throughout the meditation, you will begin noticing more and more calming experiences in your day-to-day life.

Spend a Day in Silence

If you're up for a challenge, one powerful way to experience more rest and relaxation is to spend a day in silence. This means no speaking, no one else speaking to you, no phone calls, no TV, no listening to the radio, audiobooks, videos, or podcasts—total silence!

We've grown so accustomed to stimulation overload that sitting in silence will probably feel very uncomfortable, almost eerie! But constantly hearing noise, even if it's only background noise, is still expending your energy, even if you don't really notice it. Taking a break from all noise will give your mind a chance to rest, recharge, and replenish some mental energy!

If you live with others, this can make it quite challenging to spend a day in silence, so planning your day of silence ahead of time is key to making sure people are aware of your intention. Hopefully they will honor and respect your wishes and be cooperative. You can even invite them to join you! Try to plan your day of silence when you aren't working, since attempting this activity on a workday would only bring even greater challenges!

It would be a perfect day to stay home and engage in other relaxing activities.

Participate in Community Events

Participating in community events can be very fulfilling and help you feel more deeply connected to your community. Choose community events that feel aligned with your interests and resonate with you.

You can check your local newspapers or check a community website to see what events are scheduled. If none of them really interests you, you could create your own event! Community potlucks are incredible opportunities to share nourishing food with others and connect with other souls. Community yoga and meditation classes are perfect events to practice restful and relaxing activities and connect with others.

You can also look for clubs in your community that you can join. What are your favorite hobbies? What do you want more of in your life? If you want to make more time for soothing exercise, look for walking clubs. If your goal is to learn something new, perhaps try a cooking class.

Before you attend the event, get yourself in a good headspace. Meditate if you need to, or do some deep breathing. Create the positive energy you want to attract. This will ensure you will show up as your best self and will be able to fully connect with others and enjoy all aspects of engaging with your community.

Donate

Want to make a difference? Donate to a cause or an organization that you feel called to support! Donating leads to optimistic feelings and a more positive outlook on life, which in turn makes you more grateful and peaceful.

Think about what social issues you feel connected to that you would be proud to support. Make a list of the top charities you want to contribute to as a starting point. Although donations certainly can be monetary, there are many other ways to contribute that don't include money. You can also donate material items such as food, clothing, household items, personal items, and so much more.

If you're able to, personally drop off the goods to the organization you feel called to support. You'll be able to see firsthand how your contributions are making an impact. It's a great way to feel a sense of fulfillment and like you're making a difference, because you are!

When you give to an organization in need, you'll likely experience an array of emotions, including genuine appreciation for everything you have and gratitude for being able to help others. This will be a good time to sit back and relax and reflect on all the blessings in your life, big and small alike!

Talk to a Mentor

If you're finding it hard to make time for rest in your life, you can seek out a mentor for guidance. Mentorship can reduce the stress you feel from having to figure it all out on your own. Mentors serve as advisors to less experienced people in a certain field. A good mentor wants the best for you and can open your eyes to various possibilities in your life.

Having a mentor help you with a particular goal can provide clarity and support. Connecting with others and discussing life situations can bring more awareness to our lives. Mentors aren't therapists, but a positive support system you can learn from. They can give you advice if you ask for it, and guide you through something they've personally had experience with.

Having someone to turn to if you have a question about business, relationships, career, spirituality, health, or anything else can be comforting.

You can find a mentor through a professional connection or by joining a mentorship program. When you find a mentor that you connect with, tell them your goals, including less stress and more relaxation. Together, you'll be able to create positive changes!

Get Into Bonsai

Is your physical environment in need of some calming energy? Place a bonsai plant in the room where you spend most of your time. People believe bonsai is a spiritually symbolic plant, as it symbolizes harmony and balance in nature. Bonsai exudes calm energy that relieves stress. Bonsai plants are a great way to appreciate nature and the world around you. They're calming to look at while bringing positive energy into your home.

Bonsai is the ancient art of creating miniature replicas of trees based on horticulture techniques. Artists control the trees' growth by pinching the buds, limiting fertilizer, trimming branches, and wiring stems. Caring for a bonsai tree will teach you to practice more patience and love.

Bonsai has been around for thousands of years and is a profoundly symbolic Japanese art form inspired by the Chinese art of penjing. The Japanese culture and way of life also incorporates the aspects of minimalism, peace, and harmony.

To purchase a bonsai for your home, go to a local plant store. Tune in to the tree's energy by feeling its vibration to decide which one is perfect for you. Enjoy all the peace this plant will bring to your life!

Learn Tarot Reading

Do you need guidance in a specific area of your life? Tarot readings can help! Tarot cards are a form of spiritual guidance that connects you to your inner knowing. Tarot cards can help you find clarity, develop a deeper connection with your own inner being as well as with the universe, and be an enjoyable and relaxing way to find inner peace.

Seventy-eight cards make up the tarot deck, each with its own image, message, and meaning. There are twenty-two Major Arcana cards in the deck about life's spiritual lessons. There are fifty-six Minor Arcana cards, representing daily experiences in life. Some people believe that the tarot deck contains all the spiritual lessons we encounter in life.

Whether or not you believe in the accuracy of tarot cards initially, you may be surprised by how accurate the guidance you receive feels. Many nonbelievers are converted to believers after a single reading because of how eerily precise their reading is.

It will take time to familiarize yourself with your deck of tarot cards, to learn about the meanings behind all the symbols, and to learn how to use them to do readings, so be patient and have fun with it.

Burn Incense

Would you like to create a peaceful atmosphere quickly? Burn incense! It can be an instant mood booster. We are spiritually stimulated by incense. Using incense not only produces a pleasant smell, but also calms the mind. Use incense during prayer, meditation, yoga, or whenever you want to rest.

These thin sticks are usually made of tree resin, essential oils and scents, and herbs. Incense scented with essential oils can reduce anxiety and stress. It can cleanse the air of negative energy and infuse sacred energy into a space.

Get cozy on the couch with a soft blanket, a book, a cup of coffee or tea, and the incense scent of your choice. Escape your worries by lighting incense sticks of sandalwood, jasmine, rose, lavender, or frankincense fragrances.

Use a lighter to light the bottom of the stick until you see a small flame. Let the flame burn for a moment and then blow it out. Incense sticks should not be left unattended when burning. They can burn for about thirty minutes. If you are using incense for a shorter period and you want to stop the incense from burning, simply cut off the tip of the stick with metal scissors.

Learn to Play an Instrument

Creating beautiful sounds for yourself and for others to hear is rewarding and gets you in touch with your spiritual side. Music is the universal language that can connect you with others in the world, regardless of your native language or background. No matter what genre you enjoy most, the instrument's vibrations will touch your spirit. This is a beautiful moment that helps you relax and unwind.

The first step in playing music is to learn how to read music. Don't stress, though. It is a simple process that will get easier and make more sense in time. Go to the library and find a book on reading music, watch videos online, or sign up for music lessons with a teacher. If you already know how to read music, you can skip this step or just refresh your memory.

Next is the fun part! Pick the instrument you want to learn to play. Try different instruments and see which resonates with you the most. Which one do you enjoy playing? What instrument moves you? Whether you rent or buy an instrument, embrace every step of learning a new instrument and creating music for yourself and others.

Sing with a Group

Singing is a joyful activity. Singing in a group makes it even more rewarding! The spiritual experience of singing is enhanced when a group of people sing together. The same sense of belonging and connectedness people experience from team sports is experienced when singing with a group of people. Your mind will feel less stressed and worried when you are singing because it will require you to focus on the present moment.

Whether you can sing well or not, you will still benefit from singing with others. The act of singing lowers cortisol (stress hormone) and releases endorphins and oxytocin, leading to feelings of relaxation and happiness. And being part of a group can help relieve feelings of loneliness, depression, and anxiety.

Want to find a singing group but don't know where to begin? Sing with your family, sing in a local choir, attend a concert, go to a music festival, or even sing karaoke with friends!

If you want to practice singing before becoming part of a group, consider taking voice lessons with a teacher or find free classes online. Remember, singing with a group is meant to reduce stress and promote more relaxation in your life.

Go Stargazing

There is something special about looking into the night sky full of stars. You might feel like it gives you a fresh perspective on life! A night sky lit by stars is calming and enlightening. You may be able to forget about your worries by looking at the stars and planets, even for a brief moment.

When you're stargazing, your eyes are focused on the night sky, reminding you that you live on Earth, surrounded by a vast universe. When you are aware of the universe that surrounds you, you are more mindful of your own soul. You realize that there is a huge world around you and that you are only a tiny part of it. This brings the realization that your day-to-day problems are small compared to the big world around you. This becomes a grounding and peaceful experience.

Set up a space outdoors where you can sit and observe the sky. Bring blankets, pillows, snacks, and drinks to make the experience cozy and fun. You can spend as much time as you like admiring the beautiful night sky, whether by yourself or with friends. This is just another relaxing way to experience your innate connection with nature.

Create a Sacred Space

To maximize the benefits you receive from adding more rest and relaxation into your life, it really needs to become a consistent practice. One way to encourage this new daily habit is to create a sacred space in your home dedicated to rest and relaxation. If you have a designated space devoted to helping you relax and recharge, it will give you something to look forward to, especially after a stressful day!

Your sacred space can be a corner of a room or an entire room; it's up to you! Let the other members of your household know that you are not to be disturbed when you are in your sacred space. Over time, they will see that you are much happier and calmer and that everyone benefits from your having more time to rest and relax.

Decorate your sacred space with things that make your soul happy, such as cozy blankets and pillows, books, a yoga mat, candles, plants, and anything else that promotes good feelings. This is your sacred space that you can retreat to whenever you need to take a break, or just want some me time to rest, relax your mind, or unwind with a calming meditation!

Cleanse Your Space

Smoke cleansing is an ancient spiritual ritual in which you burn dried sage leaves and use the smoke to clear negative energy, purify your space, enhance intuition, boost positive thinking, reduce stress, and promote relaxation.

You can purchase a smoke cleansing stick (dried sage in a bundle) and a heatproof bowl online or in a wellness shop. To cleanse your space: Open a window to allow the smoke and any negative energy to escape. Then set an intention for what you hope to achieve. Would you like more peace, less stress, or increased positive energy in your home? Next, evenly light the top of the bundle of sage over the heatproof bowl and let it burn for approximately ten seconds before blowing it out. It will continue to emit smoke. Carry the smoking stick around your house and swirl it around, helping the smoke to circulate all through the space, holding the bowl under it to catch any ash.

When finished, be sure to fully extinguish the smoke stick by dabbing the lit end in ash. When it has thoroughly cooled, it should be stored in a cool, dry area away from the sun. Smoke cleanse your space regularly to promote peace and relaxation!

Practice Alternate Nostril Breathing

Alternate nostril breathing is a type of breath work where you breathe through one nostril at a time. Just a few minutes of practicing this breathing technique will help you feel more relaxed.

1. Sit cross-legged with your spine tall and your facial muscles relaxed. Close your eyes and take a few deep belly breaths, and then return your breath to its natural flow.
2. Bring your right hand up to your face. Relax your index and middle fingers on the bridge of your nose. You will use your thumb to gently close the right nostril and your ring finger to close the left nostril throughout the practice.
3. To start the breath work, exhale fully and start by closing your right nostril with your right thumb. Inhale through your left nostril, close the left nostril with your ring finger, and release your thumb from your right nostril so you can fully exhale. Inhale through the right nostril, close it with your thumb, and lift your ring finger to exhale through the left nostril. Keep repeating this pattern. It will become natural to you.

Spend about five minutes practicing alternate nostril breathing, and notice how calm and balanced you feel physically and mentally after practicing.

Set a Daily Intention

Change requires awareness and intentional action. Setting a daily intention each morning is a simple practice in which you bring awareness to your own thoughts and actions and make a commitment to yourself to intend on making the day ahead a positive one.

It's as simple as just pausing for a moment and thinking about what you want to experience that day. How do you want to feel? How do you want to show up in the world? What kind of energy do you want to attract?

Simply complete the following statement: Today, I intend to _____ .

Some examples might be:

✱ Be present in the moment as much as possible
✱ Focus on feeling good
✱ Be my most authentic self
✱ Spread love and kindness wherever I go
✱ Be on time

Write your intention on a sticky note and put it somewhere you will see it repeatedly throughout the day, or set a reminder on your phone to go off several times throughout the day to remind you of your daily intention and mindfully focus on it as much as possible.

Deciding how you want to experience life and intentionally practicing this is a much more relaxing and peaceful way to live.

Take a Musical Trip Down Memory Lane

Ponder some of the happiest times in your life. Maybe you remember old family vacations, certain experiences from your school years such as school dances or sporting events, and so on. You most likely can remember certain songs that were popular during those times. Even if you can't remember any specific song titles, you most likely know what genre of music you listened to around that time and can easily search for playlists from that era.

Take some time to just lie back and relax and listen to some old songs from your past. Listening to music that you enjoyed at an earlier time in your life can be a very soothing and uplifting experience. If you really allow yourself to be present and connect with the music, you will very likely begin to experience nostalgia, which, for some, is a sort of spiritual meditation.

Nostalgia is a sentimentality for the past, typically for a period or place with positive personal associations, and has been found to lead to increases in positivity, self-esteem, confidence, resilience, hope, and optimism about the future. Nostalgia has also been found to reduce stress. Deliberately creating a nostalgic experience is a wonderful way to rest and relax.

Practice Yoga Nidra

Yoga Nidra is a form of guided meditation, a method of Pratyahara (withdrawal of senses) that allows you to tap in to a state of relaxed consciousness as the mind settles in a place between wakefulness and sleep. A typical Yoga Nidra class is thirty to forty-five minutes long, and the entire time you're lying on your back in Savasana Pose (legs extended, arms by your sides with palms facing up).

You'll be guided through the progressive movement of your awareness as you scan different parts of your body. The process allows your brain to transition from an active state of beta waves into an alpha state, the brain wave frequency that links conscious thought with the subconscious mind. Serotonin is released in this alpha state, which helps you reach a transformational experience of inner calm. The body relaxes into stillness and a deep feeling of tranquility. The brain will then begin to emit delta waves, mimicking what happens when you enter a deep, restful sleep. The difference between deep sleep and Yoga Nidra is that you stay awake during this final phase in a state of blissful relaxed consciousness.

You can also find Yoga Nidra classes online and follow along from home!

about the author

Stephanie Thomas is a certified personal trainer, health coach, and yoga teacher who believes that creating the happy, healthy life you want can be a laid-back, realistic, and, most important, restful experience. The founder of Stephanie Thomas Fitness and the creator of *The Bridal Body Workout Guide*, Stephanie's writing on health, fitness, and wellness has appeared on sites like *mindbodygreen* and *Thrive Global*. In her spare time, you can find Stephanie reading the latest health book, spending time in nature, or taking a walk with her two cavalier pups. Learn more at StephanieThomasFitness.com.